ANTONIO F. CORNO ▍ **Congenital Heart Defects**

Decision Making for Cardiac Surgery

Volume 1   Common Defects

Dedicated to my loved children
Federica, Laura and Jonathan

ANTONIO F. CORNO

Congenital Heart Defects

Decision Making for Cardiac Surgery

Volume 1   Common Defects

Foreword by LUDWIG K. VON SEGESSER

With 123 Figures in 296 Separate Illustrations

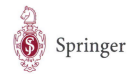

Springer

ANTONIO F. CORNO, MD, FRCS, FETCS
Department of Cardiovascular Surgery
Centre Hospitalier Universitaire Vaudois (CHUV)
46, rue du Bugnon
CH-1011 Lausanne, Switzerland

ISBN 3-7985-1415-1 Steinkopff Verlag Darmstadt

Cataloging-in-Publication Data applied for
A catalog record for this book is available from the Library of Congress.
Bibliographic information published by Die Deutsche Bibliothek
Die Deutsche Bibliothek lists this publication in the Deutsche Nationalbibliografie;
detailed bibliographic data is available in the Internet at <http://dnb.ddb.de>.

Steinkopff Verlag Darmstadt
a member of Springer Science+Business Media GmbH

http://www.steinkopff.springer.de

© Steinkopff Verlag Darmstadt 2003
Printed in Germany

Medical Editor: Sabine Ibkendanz   Production: K. Schwind
Cover Design: E. Kirchner, Heidelberg
Typesetting: K+V Fotosatz GmbH, Beerfelden

SPIN 10926437   85/7231-5 4 3 2 1 0 – Printed on acid-free paper

Foreword

Nature has the very special property to reproduce itself in unlimited variations. That is the main reason why we are all somewhat different from each other, and it is considered by some, as one of the essential faculties that allows for continuous evolution. However, natural differentiation can go a little bit and sometimes even too far. Occasionally, as one of the results, all sorts of congenital heart defects do occur in a multitude of expressions and combinations. It is interesting to note here that relatively minor congenital heart defects can become rapidly quite symptomatic and are therefore readily recognized and treated. On the other hand, major defects can appear almost compensated, and may remain hidden for a long time until secondary changes can preclude a usually promising therapeutic approach.

Phenomena such as those described can become a major issue for patients with congenital heart defects, their families, and their doctors. In an ideal world, the diagnosis of congenital heart defects should be made before birth, and the same holds true for the therapeutic strategy which can be established before delivery, in order to be able to provide the best possible care at birth if necessary, or for a more futuristic scenario even in utero whenever possible. However, for the time being, such an early approach is far from being the standard on a global scale, and the major number of patients with congenital heart defects are still referred relatively late to institutions with the required expertise for adequate diagnostics, initial treatment, and follow-up.

Access, or better, lack of access to appropriate medical facilities is certainly the predominant problem in this respect for remote areas. But even in the urban environment, where many of us do live, there are patients in need of adequate care despite the fact that the necessary facilities exist, and the social security system is set up to bear the cost generated. This somewhat surprising situation has certainly various reasons. One plausible explanation is that the great variability of congenital malformations did not allow until now to have for all these different diagnoses well-established protocols for diagnostics, and also so for treatment and decision making.

The list of diagnoses established by the European Society of Pediatric Cardiology lists 2000 congenital cardiac diagnoses, which can occur isolated or combined. Even the short list has about 100 positions, which all deserve careful attention. To make things more complicated, the presence of congenital heart disease does not preclude other malformations, and therefore even so called simple congenital heart defects can, in combination with other diseases, become a major therapeutic and decision making challenge.

"Congenital Heart Defects – Decision Making for Surgery" by Antonio Corno fills a critical gap in the currently available literature, where the diagnostic process for patients with congenital heart disease, the potential treatments, the work-up for surgery, the pre-procedural issues, and the outcome are usually reported separately. As a matter of fact, it is the integration of all that knowledge outlined above, in conjunction with the socio-cultural background of each individual patient, large or small, that allows the reader to reach a balanced view, and to determine the optimal personal therapeutic strategy. Based on his long professional experience as a pediatric cardiac surgeon dedicated to clinical practice, research, and teaching in this field, Antonio Corno has compiled all the necessary information required for successful *Decision Making for Surgery* in patients with *Congenital Heart Defects*, both, common and less common!

Lausanne, Switzerland, July 2003   Ludwig K. von Segesser

Preface

There is certainly no lack in the amount of literature covering congenital heart defects.

However, as a paediatric cardiac surgeon I am aware that on a practical level a more integrative approach taking into account the expertise of the relevant specialties is the daily bread of our profession. From tasks appearing superficially simple to most challenging decisions, each patient concerned by congenital heart malformation deserves the specialists' full attention in the context of a multidimensional cardiac, social and human situation. The author of this book feels the need for a manual attempting to bring together at least the various medical and surgical issues.

Expressly created to assist with decision-making for surgical treatment of congenital heart defects, this new reference covers all relevant aspects. The congenital heart defects are presented with each chapter devoted to a single malformation, with incidence, morphology, associated anomalies, pathophysiology, diagnosis (including clinical pattern, electrocardiogram, chest X-ray, echocardiogram, cardiac catheterization with angiography), indications for surgical treatment, details of surgical treatment, potential complications and literature references.

Morphology, pathophysiology and surgical treatment of the defects are explained with schematic drawings, while images taken from morphologic specimens, echocardiographic and angiographic investigations as well as from intra-operative photographs illustrate better than any words the key points of the decision making process for the surgical treatment of congenital heart defects.

From the long list of known heart malformations the more common defects are the focus of this first volume. One has to start with something finally, regardless the fact that infrequent defects may be far more challenging for obvious reasons. Those malformations missing in this volume will be extensively treated in a second one which is in preparation to be published in the Summer of 2004.

Lausanne, Switzerland, July 2003 ANTONIO F. CORNO

Acknowledgments

Since this book is the result of my personal experience, I would like to thank all the individuals who contributed to developing my knowledge in the field of congenital heart defects.

Acknowledgment begins with all the sick children and their families encountered during my professional life.

Then to all the teachers who contributed to my professional training, colleagues, nurses and technicians met during my career: from everybody I have learned something, from most I learned how, when and what to do in the presence of a child with a congenital heart defect; from others what should not be done which is also extremely important.

▌ **Morphology:** Thanks to the endless enthusiasm of Gaetano Thiene and his huge specimen collection at the University of Padova, where I received the rudiments of the morphology of congenital heart defects; he spent a tremendous amount of time and effort teaching the anatomy of the most frequent cardiac malformations.

While in Amsterdam for my surgical training, Anton E. Becker, another outstanding cardiac pathologist came into the operating room, scrubbed with the surgeons, explained the details of the intra-cardiac morphology and provided precious suggestions for surgical repair.

Impossible not to mention are Robert H. Anderson and Richard van Praagh for their educational books and articles as well workshops with practical demonstrations. Robert H. Anderson supported the production of this book and provided substantial input for the preparation of a few chapters.

▌ **Pathophysiology:** Understanding the pathophysiology is essential in the process of decision making for congenital heart defects. At the University of California, Los Angeles, Jay M. Jarmakani and particularly William F. Friedman were always available to explain the myocardial function in normal and sick children. Particularly important were the lessons repeatedly learned from Abraham M. Rudolph, with both editions of his remarkable book and numerous outstanding papers.

▌ **Clinical pattern:** Piero Fancini, in Milan, explained cardiac murmurs, electrocardiograms and chest X-rays, Filippo Casolo taught the basics of angiocardiography. Tom G. Losekoot continued this education in Amsterdam on hemodynamics, followed by Roberta G. Williams at the University of California, Los Angeles, on pre-operative and post-operative echocardiography and

Joseph K. Perloff on the problems of the growing population of adults with congenital heart defects.

A substantial part of my knowledge on clinical problems has been acquired by daily practice, particularly in the pediatric hospital "Bambino Gesú", Rome, which all the pediatric cardiologists contributed to, particularly Bruno Marino and Salvatore Giannico. A similar positive experience occurred years later in Glasgow, with Neil Wilson.

∎ **Surgery:** The beginning of my training was at the University of Padova, with the late Vincenzo Gallucci, who taught me how to repair an atrioventricular septal defect and a tetralogy of Fallot.

Further important progress was the exposure to daily practice with Carlo Marcelletti, not only in surgery but also in pre-operative evaluation as well as in post-operative care. Most of the intra-operative photographs of this book have been taken during the period spent with him.

Other surgeons substantially contributed to improving my surgical expertise:
∎ Hillel Laks, at the University of California, Los Angeles, who was very demanding and meticulous.
∎ Yves Lecompte, in Paris, thanks to his straightforward style, corrected when needed, before actually teaching how surgery should be done and sometimes how to be inventive. His essential observation was that "every patient is unique".
∎ Ludwig K. von Segesser, my current Chairman, is one of the few remaining surgeons able to operate on a neonate of 2 kg with transposition of the great arteries and single coronary artery, a 86 year-old patient with the rupture of a thoraco-abdominal aneurysm and to support the decision for a Ross operation on a young adult with 4 previous sternotomies. Not to mention his constant intellectual curiosity to develop new techniques and tools in the research laboratory before clinical application. He also pushed me, more than anyone else, to complete this book.

Other surgeons participated in extending my surgical knowledge during meetings and workshops, like all the colleagues of the European Congenital Heart Surgeons Foundation.

Other contributions came from the visits to the hospitals of Aldo R. Castañeda, Mark R. de Leval, Richard A. Jonas, William I. Norwood, Lucio Parenzan, Claude Planché, Jan M. Quaegebeur, Jaroslav Stark and Pascal Vouhé.

∎ **Cardiopulmonary bypass:** Yves Durandy, in Paris, demonstrated that cardiopulmonary bypass can and should be performed in a way very similar to the physiological conditions.

∎ **Post-operative care:** I learned from all the colleagues and nurses in the pediatric hospital "Bambino Gesú", Roma.

Yves Durandy proved that the post-operative period should respect closely the physiological conditions with the fewest medications and interventions.

Leonardo Milella, in Glasgow, confirmed that it is possible for the anesthesist and surgeon to collaborate very well in the post-operative care, with evident advantage for the patients.

▮ **Research:** Several individuals were very important in different periods of my experience with experimental and clinical research, but none as much as Gerald D. Buckberg, University of California, Los Angeles, who played a pivotal role in teaching the methodology of research.

Philippe Clavel, Lausanne, contributed to this book with the graphics and a lot of patience with my requests.

Special thanks to Bruno Marino, a friend before being a pediatric cardiologist in Rome, who very kindly reviewed the text of this book and contributed several illustrations.

A profession constitutes only a part of our life: I deeply acknowledge my family's unconditional support, particularly for my wife Josie's patience for the long hours I spent at nights and week-ends working to complete this book.

Lausanne, Switzerland, July 2003   ANTONIO F. CORNO

Table of Contents

CHAPTER 1.1 Total anomalous pulmonary venous connection

▮ Incidence

Anomalous pulmonary venous connection is the 15th most common congenital heart defect (1.4% of all congenital heart defects).

▮ Morphology

All the pulmonary veins connect anomalously to the right atrium, either directly or via the coronary sinus, superior vena cava, or inferior vena cava; a patent foramen ovale or atrial septal defect allows mixed blood in the right atrium to enter the left heart for systemic distribution; usually the confluence of the pulmonary veins is posterior to the left atrium, but separate from it.

There are four basic types:

- ▮ Supracardiac: the anomalous connection is to an ascending vertical vein, usually on the left and connected to the left innominate vein; pulmonary venous obstruction is possible;
- ▮ Cardiac: the pulmonary veins connect directly to the right atrium or (more frequently) to the coronary sinus; pulmonary venous obstruction is rare;
- ▮ Infracardiac (or infradiaphragmatic): the connection is to intraabdominal veins (more frequently to the portal vein); pulmonary venous obstruction is very frequent;
- ▮ Mixed: the entire pulmonary venous drainage is through two (or more) of the above connections.

▮ Associated anomalies

Ventricular septal defect, patent ductus arteriosus, cor triatriatum, aortic coarctation, aortic arch interruption, aortic stenosis, pulmonary stenosis; very rare is the association with conotruncal malformations: tetralogy of Fallot, transposition of the great arteries, double outlet right ventricle; frequent is the presence in patients with situs ambiguus and/or (right) atrial isomerism.

▮ Pathophysiology

Total left-to-right shunt, with volume overload of the right heart, and increased pulmonary blood flow; right-to-left shunt at the atrial level, with poor left ventricular filling in case (rare) of restrictive interatrial communication; pulmonary venous congestion and pulmonary hypertension (often at the suprasystemic level) in case of obstructed pulmonary venous connection.

Following birth, pulmonary vascular resistance drops sharply, and pulmonary blood flow increases. Increased pulmonary blood flow due to total anomalous pulmonary venous return in the absence of pulmonary venous obstruction results in an increased return of blood to the anomalous pulmonary venous drainage, and hence flow back to the right atrium and right ventricle; depending on the presence and degree of right-to-left shunting at the atrial level, left ventricular output is either maintained or decreased, while right ventricular output is greatly increased.

The ductus arteriosus may remain patent for days or weeks after birth, particularly in infants hypoxic with pulmonary venous obstruction. If the pulmonary vascular resistance is very high, blood will shunt from the pulmonary artery to the aorta, effectively stealing blood from the pulmonary circulation and rendering the baby even more cyanotic. Conversely, if the resistance is reversed, the direction of shunting will also be reversed. Arterial-level or ventricular-level shunting, the latter occurring in the presence of a ventricular septal defect, in conditions of high pulmonary vascular resistance may occasionally be important in maintaining systemic blood flow, particularly when the left atrium and left ventricle are hypoplastic or the patent foramen ovale restrictive.

▌ Diagnosis

▌ **Clinical pattern:** unobstructed form: similar to an atrial septal defect with large left-to-right shunt, with moderate heart failure usually in the first year of life, failure to thrive, poor feeding, and recurrent chest infections; obstructed form: severe heart failure and/or cyanosis, poor peripheral perfusion, respiratory insufficiency, tachypnea (usually in the first month of life).

▌ **Electrocardiogram:** right axis deviation, right atrial hypertrophy, right ventricular hypertrophy.

▌ **Chest X-ray:** unobstructed form: moderate cardiomegaly, with increased pulmonary vascularity; obstructed form: pulmonary edema, absent cardiomegaly; wide upper mediastinum (snowman sign) more frequently in older infants and children with supracardiac type.

▌ **Echocardiogram:** right ventricular diastolic overload, pulmonary artery dilatation, echo free space posterior to the left atrium; relative hypoplasia of the left heart; definitive diagnosis in most of the cases with color

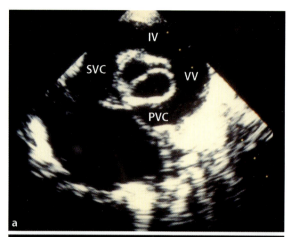

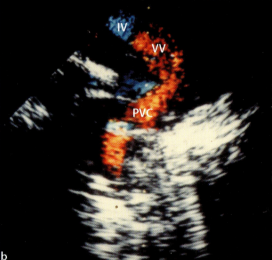

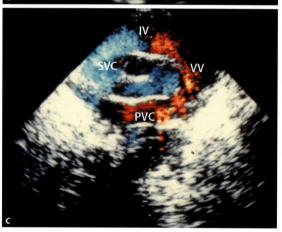

Fig. 1.1.1. Total anomalous pulmonary venous connection. **a** echocardiography showing supracardiac type, **b** color Doppler echocardiography showing supracardiac type, **c** color Doppler echocardiography showing supracardiac type. Subsequent imaging (*IV* innominate vein, *PVC* pulmonary venous collector, *SVC* superior vena cava, *VV* vertical vein)

flow Doppler, with identification of all the pulmonary veins, the venous connection to the systemic circulation (Fig. 1.1.1), the site of obstruction, the presence of pulmonary hypertension and associated lesions.

■ **Cardiac catheterization:** limited to the cases with:
■ suspect of mixed type of anomalous connection,
■ suspect of associated complex malformations,
■ morphology of all pulmonary veins not identified with echocardiography (Figs. 1.1.2, 1.1.3 and 1.1.4).

■ Indications for surgical treatment

Obstructed form: emergency surgery at any age, possibly based on echo only; balloon atrial septostomy is occasionally beneficial in cases of a restrictive patent foramen ovale, which may improve left ventricular filling, ameliorate features of low cardiac output and decrease pulmonary venous pressure.

Unobstructed form: elective surgical treatment, in infancy; in childhood, surgical treatment once pulmonary vascular obstructive disease is excluded.

■ Surgical treatment (on cardiopulmonary bypass)

Surgical repair, generally reported with deep hypothermia and circulatory arrest, can be performed not only in children, but also in infants, with continuous perfusion, therefore avoiding circulatory arrest.

■ **Supracardiac and infracardiac type:** a large anastomosis is created between the anterior wall of the common pulmonary venous sinus and the posterior wall of the left atrium, both widely opened to obtain an unrestrictive connection; the approach can be biatrial (right atriotomy, opening of the interatrial

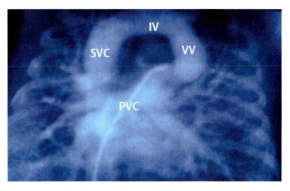

Fig. 1.1.2. Total anomalous pulmonary venous connection. Angiography showing supracardiac type (*IV* innominate vein, *PVC* pulmonary venous collector, *SVC* superior vena cava, *VV* vertical vein)

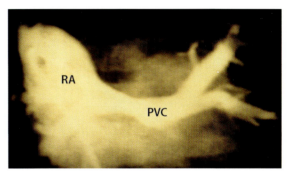

Fig. 1.1.3. Total anomalous pulmonary venous connection. Angiography showing cardiac type: pulmonary venous connection to the right atrium (*PVC* pulmonary venous collector, *RA* right atrium)

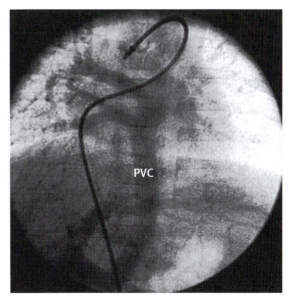

Fig. 1.1.4. Total anomalous pulmonary venous connection. Angiography showing infradiaphragmatic type (*PVC* pulmonary venous collector)

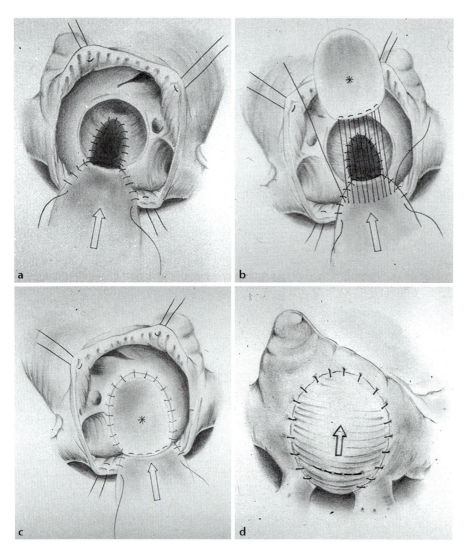

Fig. 1.1.5. Total anomalous pulmonary venous connection: surgery. Double patch technique: **a** anastomosis of the pulmonary venous collector to the opened atrial wall and to the external pericardial patch (arrow = external pericardial patch), **b** suture of the internal Teflon patch to the internal aspect of the pericardial patch, in a position higher than the interatrial septum, in order to enlarge the left atrium (asterisk = internal Teflon patch, arrow = external pericardial patch), **c** completed suture of the internal Teflon patch (new interatrial septum) to the pericardial patch (asterisk = internal Teflon patch, arrow = exteral pericardial patch), **d** completed suture of the external pericardial patch (arrow = external pericardial patch). (Reproduced with permission from: Corno AF, Giamberti A, Carotti A, Giannico S, Marino B, Marcelletti C (1990) Total anomalous pulmonary venous connection: surgical repair with a "double patch" technique. Ann Thorac Surg 49:492–494)

septum), posterior or superior (between aorta, right pulmonary artery and the roof of the left atrium); the ascending (or descending) vertical vein may be left open (to allow heart decompression), or ligated, or transected and opened longitudinally to be utilized to create a wider anastomosis; the patent foramen ovale may be closed or left (partially) open to allow heart decompression; the left atrium may be enlarged with a single or double patch technique (Fig. 1.1.5), to improve left ventricular filling.

■ **Cardiac type:** the total pulmonary venous return is deviated to the left atrium through an unrestricted (or surgically enlarged) interatrial communication by a patch; in the case of coronary sinus type, the roof of the coronary sinus is incised (or excised) to create an unrestricted connection.

∎ **Mixed type:** surgical treatment must be individualized and based on the particular morphology.

∎ Potential complications

Acute pulmonary edema, pulmonary arterial hypertensive crisis, phrenic nerve damage, pulmonary venous obstruction, anastomotic obstruction, residual or recurrent intra-atrial shunt, supraventricular arrhythmias.

∎ References

Amodeo A, Corno AF, Marino B, Carta MG, Marcelletti C (1990) Combined repair of transposed great arteries and total anomalous pulmonary venous connection. Ann Thorac Surg 50:820–821

Bove EL, de Leval MR, Taylor JFN, Macartney FJ, Szarnicki RJ, Stark J (1981) Infradiaphragmatic total anomalous pulmonary venous drainage: surgical treatment and long-term results. Ann Thorac Surg 31:544

Corno AF, Giamberti A, Carotti A, Giannico S, Marino B, Marcelletti C (1990) Total anomalous pulmonary venous connection: surgical repair with a "double patch" technique. Ann Thorac Surg 49:492–494

Corno AF (1997) An unusual type of total anomalous pulmonary venous connection. Ann Thorac Surg 64:1218

Corno AF, von Segesser LK (1999) Is hypothermia necessary in pediatric cardiac surgery? Eur J Cardiothorac Surg 15:110–111

Corno AF (2000) Surgery for congenital heart disease. Curr Opinion Cardiol 15:238–243

Ferencz C, Rubin JD, McCarter RJ (1985) Congenital heart disease: prevalence at livebirth. The Baltimore-Washington infant study. Am J Epidemiol 121:31–36

Freedom RM, Olley PM, Coceani F, Rowe RD (1978) The prostaglandin challenge. Test to unmask obstructed total anomalous pulmonary venous connection in asplenia syndrome. Br Heart J 40:91–94

Fyler DC, Buckley LP, Hellenbrand WE, Cohn HE (1980) Report of the New England regional infant care program. Pediatrics 65(Suppl):375–461

Giamberti A, Corno AF, Nava S, Amoeo A, Giannico S, Marino B, Marcelletti C (1989) Connessione venosa polmonare anomala totale: trattamento chirurgico. Arch Chir Tor Cardiovasc 11:23

Gomes MMR, Feldt RH, McGoon DC, Danielson GK (1970) Total anomalous pulmonary venous connection: surgical considerations and results of operation. J Thorac Cardiovasc Surg 60:116

Goor DA, Yellin A, Frand M, Smolinsky A, Neufeldt H (1966) The operative problem of small left atrium in total anomalous pulmonary venous connection: report of 5 patients. Ann Thorac Surg 72:245

Grabitz RG, Joffres MR, Collins-Nakai RL (1988) Congenital heart disease: incidence in the first year of life. The Alberta heritage pediatric cardiology program. Am J Epidemiol 128:381–388

Hoffman JIE, Kaplan S (2002) The incidence of congenital heart disease. J Am Coll Cardiol 39:1890–1900

Hyde JA, Stumper O, Barth MJ, Wright JG, Silove ED, de Giovanni JV, Brawn WJ, Sethia B (1999) Total anomalous pulmonary venous connection: outcome of surgical correction and management of recurrent venous obstruction. Eur J Cardiothorac Surg 15:735–740

Jonas RA, Smolinsky A, Mayer JE, Castaneda AR (1987) Obstructed pulmonary venous drainage with total anomalous pulmonary venous connection to the coronary sinus. Am J Cardiol 59:431–435

Katz NM, Kirklin JW, Pacifico AD (1978) Concepts and practices in surgery for total anomalous pulmonary venous connection. Ann Thorac Surg 25:479–487

Kirshbom PM, Myung RJ, Gaynor JW, Ittenbach RF, Paridon SM, DeCampli WM, Karl TR, Spray TL (2002) Preoperative pulmonary venous obstruction affects long-term outcome for survivors of total anomalous pulmonary venous connection repair. Ann Thorac Surg 74:1616–1620

Kumar RN, Dharmapuram AK, Rao IM, Gopalakrishnan VC, Pillai VR, Nazer YA, Cartmill T (2001) The fate of the unligated vertical vein after surgical correction of total anomalous pulmonary venous connection in early infancy. J Thorac Cardiovasc Surg 122:615–617

Lacour-Gayet F, Zoghbi J, Serraf AE, Belli E, Piot D, Rey C, Marcon F, Bruniaux J, Planché C (1999) Surgical management of progressive pulmonary venous obstruction after repair of total anomalous pulmonary venous connection. J Thorac Cardiovasc Surg 117:679–687

Marino B, Corno AF, Carotti A, Pasquini L, Giannico S, Guccione P, Bevilacqua M, De Simone G, Marcelletti C (1990) Pediatric cardiac surgery guided by echocardiography. Scand J Thorac Cardiovasc Surg 24:197–201

Neill CA, Ferencz C, Sabiston C (1960) The familial occurrence of hypoplastic right lung with systemic arterial supply and venous drainage: "scimitar syndrome". Johns Hopkins Med J 107:1–20

Ootaki Y, Yamaguchi M, Oshima Y, Yoshimura N, Oka S (2001) Repair of total anomalous pulmonary venous connection without cardiopulmonary bypass. Ann Thorac Surg 72:249–251

Roe BB (1970) Posterior approach to correction of total anomalous pulmonary venous return. J Thorac Cardiovasc Surg 59:748

Sano S, Brawn WJ, Mee RBB (1989) Total anomalous pulmonary venous drainage. J Thorac Cardiovasc Surg 97:886–892

Turley K, Tucker WY, Ullyot DJ, Ebet PA (1980) Total anomalous pulmonary venous connection in infancy: influence of age and type of lesion. Am J Cardiol 45:92

Van Praagh R, Harken AH, Delisle G, Ando M, Gross RE (1972) Total anomalous pulmonary venous drainage to the coronary sinus: a revised procedure for its correction. J Thorac Cardiovasc Surg 64:132

Partial anomalous pulmonary venous connection

▌ Incidence

Anomalous pulmonary venous connection is the 15th most common congenital heart defect (1.4% of all congenital heart defects).

▌ Morphology

One or more, but not all, of the pulmonary veins are connected to the right atrium or to one or more of its tributaries.

Left-sided pulmonary veins usually connect anomalously to derivatives of the left cardinal system: coronary sinus, left innominate vein.

Anomalous right pulmonary veins usually connect to derivatives of the right cardinal system: superior vena cava, inferior vena cava or right atrium.

The most common type of partial anomalous pulmonary venous connection is the sinus venosus defect: the right upper and middle lobe pulmonary veins (right superior pulmonary vein) attach to the low superior vena cava or the superior vena cava-right atrial junction, an arrangement present in about 95% of patients with subcaval atrial septal defect.

Occasionally the entire right superior pulmonary vein connects to the superior vena cava without an associated subcaval atrial septal defect; the connection is then almost always well above (superior to) the superior vena cava-right atrial junction.

▌ **Scimitar syndrome:** all the right pulmonary veins (occasionally the middle and lower pulmonary veins) are connected to the inferior vena cava just above or below the diaphragm; the orifice of the right pulmonary veins is usually very close to the orifices of the hepatic veins.

The term 'scimitar syndrome' was first applied to a radiographic finding in a familial disease characterized by a right-sided heart with partial anomalous pulmonary venous connection; the anomalous connection was to the inferior vena cava and the shadow produced was likened to the curve of a Turkish sword.

The left innominate vein is the usual site of anomalous connection of the left pulmonary veins; uncommon sites of anomalous connection of the left pulmonary veins are coronary sinus, inferior vena cava, superior vena cava, right atrium and left subclavian vein.

The veins from the left upper lobe, or more frequently from the whole left lung, connect to the left innominate vein via a derivative of the left cardinal system; this connecting vein has been called a persistent left superior vena cava, but since it makes no direct connection to the heart, it cannot be identified as such; a preferable term is anomalous vertical vein.

Bilateral partial anomalous pulmonary venous connection (=partial anomalous venous connection of both lungs) is very rare: the most common variant is probably that in which the left superior pulmonary vein attaches to the left innominate vein by way of an anomalous vertical vein, and the right superior pulmonary vein attaches to the superior vena cava-right atrial junction.

▮ Associated anomalies

Partial anomalous pulmonary venous connection may coexist with nearly all varieties of congenital heart disease, but such cases are not considered the primary lesion unless the anomalous pulmonary venous connection is the dominant hemodynamic lesion.

The presence of an ostium secundum or fossa ovalis atrial septal defect is usual; rarely the atrial septum is intact.

Other associated anomalies include the following: ventricular septal defect, patent ductus arteriosus, pulmonary valvar stenosis and persistence of the left superior vena cava.

Scimitar syndrome is associated with various degrees of right lung hypoplasia, dextroposition of the heart; the arterial blood supply to the right lung may be via aorto-pulmonary collateral vessels from the descending thoracic aorta; occasionally, true pulmonary sequestration and/or diaphragmatic anomalies may be associated; generally the atrial septum is intact.

▮ Pathophysiology

The fundamental physiologic disturbance is similar to that in atrial septal defect: increased pulmonary blood flow as a consequence of recirculation of oxygenated blood through the lungs, with volume overload of the right heart due to the left-to-right shunt.

The factors determining the hemodynamic state include the following: the number of anomalously connected veins; the site of the anomalous connections; the presence or absence of atrial septal defect.

▮ Diagnosis

Physical examination is very similar to that in atrial septal defect.

▮ **Clinical pattern:** usually asymptomatic; rarely congestive heart failure and/or recurrent upper respiratory infections; in adults, frequently exertional dyspnea, easy fatigability, shortness of breath, arrhythmias; potential development of pulmonary hypertension with or without pulmonary vascular obstructive disease.

▮ **Electrocardiogram:** incomplete right bundle branch block; right ventricular hypertrophy in patients with pulmonary hypertension.

▮ **Chest X-ray:** moderate cardiac enlargement, with dilation of the right chambers and of the pulmonary trunk; increased pulmonary vascularity. In the scimitar syndrome the anomalous vein forms a curved shadow at the right lung base in the anteroposterior view.

▮ **Echocardiogram:** diagnostic in almost all cases, permitting the precise localization of the pulmonary vein(s) anomalously connected (Fig. 1.2.1); in uncomplicated cases, surgical decision-making can be based on echo findings alone; very useful is the Doppler color flow.

▮ **Cardiac catheterization:** a step-up in oxygen saturation is present at the site of entry of the anomalous vein(s); with contrast injection directly into the pulmonary veins, the venous phase reliably demonstrates the abnormal venous connection(s) (Fig. 1.2.2); performed in complicated cases and/or in adults with pulmonary hypertension to measure pulmonary vascular resistance and to rule out (or to quantitate the degree of) pulmonary vascular obstructive disease.

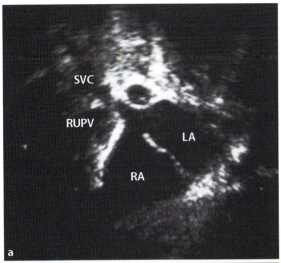

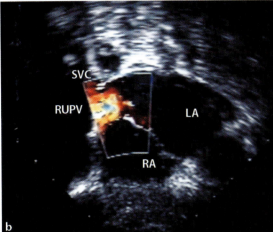

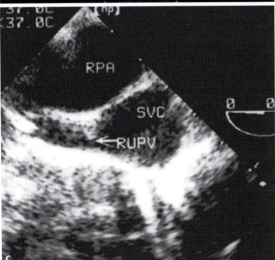

◼ Indications for surgical treatment

In the presence of an isolated partial anomalous pulmonary venous connection, the natural history generally appears comparable to that in uncomplicated atrial septal defects; therefore the indications for surgical treatment will be the same.

Asymptomatic or mild symptoms: repair at preschool age.

Severe symptoms (rarely): repair in infancy.

Adults with pulmonary hypertension: repair in absence of pulmonary vascular obstructive disease.

In asymptomatic patients with anomalous connection of only one pulmonary vein, without atrial septal defect and without other cardiac anomalies, the surgical indication may be questionable.

◼ Surgical treatment (on cardiopulmonary bypass)

◼ **Anomalous right pulmonary vein(s) connected to the superior vena cava:** The right atrial incision depends on the position of the anomalous pulmonary vein(s).

Standard oblique atriotomy: the upper right pulmonary vein is deviated to the left atrium by means of a patch (synthetic or pericardial), sewn along the wall of the superior caval vein so as to include the anomalously connected vein(s); suturing of the

Fig. 1.2.1. Partial anomalous venous connection: echocardiography. **a** short axis subcostal view showing the anomalous connection of the right upper pulmonary vein to the superior vena cava and the sinus venosus atrial septal defect (photograph courtesy of Dr. Nicole Sekarski), **b** short axis subcostal view with color Doppler showing the flow from the anomalous right upper pulmonary vein to the superior vena cava and the left-to-right shunt through the sinus venosus atrial septal defect (photograph courtesy of Dr. Nicole Sekarski), **c** transesophageal view showing the anomalous right upper pulmonary vein connected to the superior vena cava (photograph courtesy of Dr. Pierre-Guy Chassot). *LA* left atrium, *RA* right atrium, *RPA* right pulmonary artery, *RUPV* right upper pulmonary vein, *SVC* superior vena cava

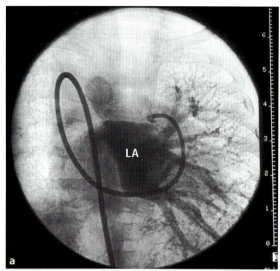

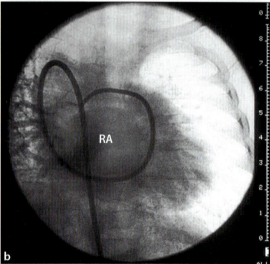

Fig. 1.2.2. Partial anomalous venous connection: angiography. **a** contrast injection into the left pulmonary artery, with venous phase showing the left pulmonary veins normally connected to the left atrium, and the sinus venosus atrial septal defect (*LA* left atrium), **b** contrast injection into the right pulmonary artery, with venous phase showing the anomalous right pulmonary veins connected to the right atrium (*RA* right atrium)

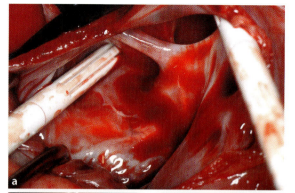

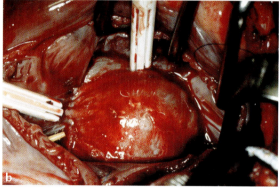

Fig. 1.2.3. Partial anomalous pulmonary venous connection in superior vena cava: surgery. **a** intra-operative photograph showing the right pulmonary veins connected to the superior vena cava and the sinus venosus atrial septal defect, **b** intra-operative photograph showing the pericardial patch deviating the right pulmonary veins into the left atrium through the atrial septal defect

patch is then carried down into the right atrium, and then sewn around an unrestricted interatrial communication (already present or surgically created) in the upper part of the interatrial septum. In this way the anomalously connected right pulmonary vein(s) could drain through a tunnel, whose posterior wall is composed of the superior caval vein and whose anterior wall is composed of

the patch, through the atrial septal defect into the left atrium (Fig. 1.2.3).

Posterior incision: another surgical option is the posterior incision of the right atrium, prolonged on the superior vena cava; this approach allows the plastic procedure enlarging the superior vena cava, by a synthetic or pericardial gusset placed in the superior vena cava-right atrial junction.

■ **Anomalous right pulmonary vein(s) connected to the inferior vena cava:** Two surgical options are available: tunneling the anomalous right pulmonary vein(s) to the left atrium through an atrial septal defect (like for the anomalous connection to the superior vena cava), or disconnection of the anomalous venous channel from the inferior vena cava and direct anastomosis to the left atrium.

■ **Anomalous left pulmonary vein(s):** Different techniques have been reported to repair the anomalous left pulmonary vein(s), all considering an end-to-side or side-to-side anastomosis between the left pulmonary vein(s) and the left auricular appendage.

The simplest surgical technique consists of a side-to-side left pulmonary vein(s) to the left atrial anastomosis, ligating the vertical vein at its junction with the innominate vein; this procedure does not require the institution of cardiopulmonary bypass and it can be performed via a left postero-lateral thoracotomy (in the absence of associated lesions).

An alternative option is the anastomosis between the left pulmonary vein(s) and the stump of the transected left auricular appendage.

Because of the potential occurrence of late stenosis, another technique has been reported consisting of a long incision in the lateral aspect of the left auricular appendage down to the left atrium; the anomalous vein is cut transversely; a T extension is then made posteriorly; the resulting end-to-side anastomosis is then very wide.

■ **Scimitar syndrome:** Correction of the scimitar syndrome may be technically demanding due to the infradiaphragmatic portion of the anomalous venous connection. Exposure of this portion of the vein is afforded by splitting the diaphragm to the veno-caval hiatus. In some patients, the repair may only require removal of the inferior vena cava cannula to expose the anomalous venous ostium during a brief period of deep hypothermic circulatory arrest. In this instance, an intra-atrial baffle is used in much the same way as a partial anomalous venous connection with a sinus venosus defect. A final alternative technique consists of extracardiac reimplantation of the scimitar vein into the posterior wall of the right atrium followed by transposition of the atrial septum anterior to the new ostium, either directly or with a patch.

■ Potential complications

Residual or recurrent atrial septal defect, air embolism (early), systemic and pulmonary thromboembolism (late), supraventricular arrhythmias, pulmonary vein(s) obstruction, vena cava obstruction.

■ References

Baron O, Roussel JC, Videcoq M, Guerin P, Gournay V, Lefevre M (2002) Partial anomalous pulmonary venous connection: correction by intra-atrial baffle and cavo-atrial anastomosis. J Card Surg 17:166–169

Corno AF, Zoia E, Santoro F, Camesasca C, Biagioli B, Grossi A (1992) Epicardial damage induced by topical cooling during pediatric cardiac surgery. Br Heart J 67:174–176

Corno AF, Rosti L, Machado I (1995) Horseshoe lung associated with anomalous pulmonary venous connection without pulmonary hypoplasia. Cardiol Young 5:91

Corno AF (1996) Bilateral partial anomalous pulmonary venous connection with intact atrial septum. Asian Cardiovasc Ann 4:181

Corno AF, von Segesser LK (1999) Is hypothermia necessary in pediatric cardiac surgery? Eur J Cardiothorac Surg 15:110–111

Da Cruz E, Milella L, Corno AF (1998) Left isomerism with tetralogy of Fallot and anomalous systemic and pulmonary venous connections. Cardiol Young 8:131–133

Fyler DC, Buckley LP, Hellenbrand WE, Cohn HE (1980) Report of the New England Regional Infant Care Program. Pediatrics 65(Suppl):375–461

Gaynor JW, Burch M, Dollery C, Sullivan ID, Deanfield JE, Elliott MJ (1995) Repair of anomalous pulmonary venous connection to the superior vena cava. Ann Thorac Surg 59:1471–1475

Grabitz RG, Joffres MR, Collins-Nakai RL (1988) Congenital heart disease: incidence in the first year of life. The Alberta heritage pediatric cardiology program. Am J Epidemiol 128:381–388

Hoffman JIE, Kaplan S (2002) The incidence of congenital heart disease. J Am Coll Cardiol 39:1890–1900

Kirklin JW, Ellis FH, Wood ED (1956) Treatment of anomalous pulmonary venous connections in association with interatrial communications. Surgery 39:389

Morgan JR, Forker AD (1971) Syndrome of hypoplasia of the right lung and dextroposition of the heart: scimitar sign with normal pulmonary venous drainage. Circulation 43:27

Murphy JW, Kerr AR, Kirklin JW (1971) Intracardiac repair for anomalous pulmonary venous connection of right lung to inferior vena cava. Ann Thorac Surg 11:38

Ports TA, Turley K, Brundage BH, Ebert PA (1979) Operative correction of total left anomalous pulmonary venous return. Ann Thorac Surg 27:246

Swan HJC, Kirklin JW, Becu LM, Wood EH (1957) Anomalous connection of right pulmonary veins to superior vena cava with interatrial communications: hemodynamic data in eight cases. Circulation 16:54

Trusler GA, Kazenelson G, Freedom RM, Williams WG, Rowe RD (1980) Late results following repair of partial anomalous pulmonary venous connection with sinus venous atrial septal defect. J Thorac Cardiovasc Surg 79:776

Warden HE, Gustafson RA, Zarnay TJ, Neal WA (1984) An alternative method for repair of partial anomalous pulmonary venous connection to the superior vena cava. Ann Thorac Surg 38:601

▍ Incidence

As an isolated lesion atrial septal defect is the 3rd most common congenital heart defect (7.7% of all congenital heart defects). However, it is seen in 33–50% of other congenital heart diseases. Secundum atrial septal defects are more common in females.

▍ Morphology (Fig. 1.3.1)

To understand the anatomy conditioning shunts between the atrial chambers, it is crucial to appreciate the difference between a defect of the atrial septum and an interatrial communication.

The atrial septum is very limited in its extent, being effectively confined to the floor of the fossa ovalis (the flap valve) and its inferior rim (separating the fossa from the coronary sinus – the sinus septum). The posterior, superior and anterior rims of the fossa (so-called "septum secundum") are, in reality, the infolded atrial walls, and not true septal structures; it is possible to pass from the right to left atrium across the superior rim, but only by first going outside the heart. It is this arrangement of septal and non-septal structures which determines the anatomy of interatrial communications.

▍ *True atrial septal defects*: defects existing within the floor of the fossa ovalis (Fig. 1.3.2); they can be produced by an insufficient or perforated flap valve; defects within the fossa (so-called "secundum" defects) must be distinguished from probe-patency of the fossa, in which the flap valve overlaps, but does not seal anatomically, the rim.

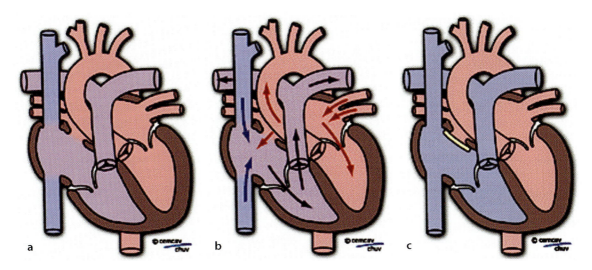

Fig. 1.3.1. Atrial septal defect ostium secundum type: **a** morphology, **b** pathophysiology, **c** surgery

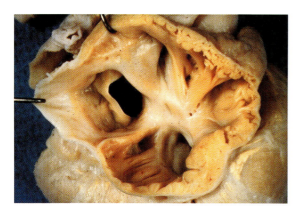

Fig. 1.3.2. Atrial septal defect ostium secundum type: morphology (photograph courtesy of Dr. Bruno Marino)

- *Sinus venosus*: interatrial communications in the mouth of usually the superior, but sometimes the inferior, vena cava; they are outside the floor of the fossa ovalis; their anatomical feature is overriding of the superior or posterior margin by the mouth of the superior or inferior vena cava, respectively.
- *Coronary sinus*: defects existing through the mouth of the sinus when there is a wide fenestration between the wall of the sinus and the left atrium; usually, but not always, the left superior vena cava drains to the roof of the left atrium (see chapter "Unroofed coronary sinus").
- *Ostium primum*: holes between the leading edge of the atrial septum and the upper margin of the ventricular septum; they are atrioventricular septal defects and have a common atrioventricular junction (see chapter "Atrioventricular septal defects").

▮ Associated anomalies

Atrial septal defects within the fossa ovalis may coexist with nearly all varieties of congenital heart disease, but such cases are not considered the primary lesion unless the left-to-right shunt at the atrial level is the dominant hemodynamic lesion.

Partial anomalous pulmonary venous connection (virtually always present in patients with sinus venosus defect), mitral valvar prolapse, ventricular septal defect, patent ductus arteriosus, pulmonary valvar stenosis, peripheral pulmonary arterial stenosis, and persistence of the left superior vena cava are the lesions which are more frequently found secondary to interatrial communications.

▮ Pathophysiology

Left-to-right shunt at the atrial level, with volume overload of the right heart and increased pulmonary blood flow. The amount of left-to-right shunt is determined by the relative compliances of left and right ventricles during diastole. The right ventricular compliance is influenced by the degree of pulmonary vascular resistance. In the neonatal period the pulmonary vascular resistance is elevated, the right ventricular compliance is decreased, and consequently there is little left-to-right shunt. As pulmonary vascular resistance decreases, the right ventricular compliance increases, and the left-to-right shunt increases. Therefore, it is very rare to find infants with an isolated atrial septal defect with intractable congestive heart failure and failure to thrive.

Factors causing increase pulmonary blood flow, and consequently early presentation include:
- Additional shunts, like ventricular septal defect, patent ductus arteriosus
- Myocardial dysfunction
- Anatomically small left ventricle
- Systemic hypertension.

Pulmonary vascular obstructive disease rarely manifests in atrial septal defect before 20 years of age. It is seen in 5–10% of adults with unrepaired atrial septal defects.

▮ Diagnosis

On examination there is a hyperactive precordium with a prominent right ventricular impulse. Auscultation reveals a prominent first heart sound. The second heart sound is split wider than normal and there is no respiratory variation since the blood flow through the pulmonary valve is always increased due to the left to right shunting at the atrial level causing a delay in pulmonary valve closure throughout the respiratory cycle. A systolic (crescendo-decrescendo) murmur is heard at the left upper sternal border, due to increase blood flow across the pulmonary valve, and in a larger atrial septal defect a diastolic early murmur at the left lower sternal border is heard, due to increase blood flow across the tricuspid valve.

■ **Clinical pattern:** usually asymptomatic; rarely congestive heart failure and/or recurrent upper respiratory infections; in adults, frequently exertional dyspnea, easy fatigability, shortness of breath, arrhythmias; potential development of pulmonary hypertension with or without pulmonary vascular obstructive disease; potential occurrence of "paradoxical" systemic embolism.

■ **Electrocardiogram:** incomplete right bundle branch block, rR in right chest leads; rarely prolonged PR interval; tall P waves suggesting right atrial enlargement.

■ **Chest X-ray:** moderate cardiomegaly, with dilation of the right chambers and of the pulmonary trunk; increased pulmonary vascularity; small aortic arch.

■ **Echocardiogram:** diagnostic in all cases (Fig. 1.3.3), permitting the distinction of true septal defects from interatrial communications (the subcostal view is the most useful); Doppler color flow (Fig. 1.3.4) shows left-to-right shunt across the atrial septal defect, unless the pulmonary vascular resistance is high resulting in higher pressure in the right atrium compared to the left atrium, leading to right-to-left shunt at the atrial level; the right atrium and right ventricle appear dilated; right ventricular dilation may lead to flattening of the interventricular septum; in adults with poor echogenic window,

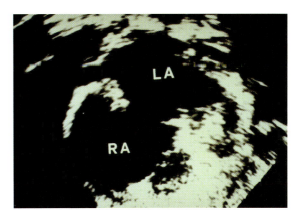

Fig. 1.3.3. Atrial septal defect: echocardiogram. Four chamber view showing the interatrial communication (*LA* left atrium, *RA* right atrium) (reproduced with permission from Marino B, Thiene G (1990) Atlante di anatomia ecocardiografica delle cardiopatie congenite, USES, Firenze)

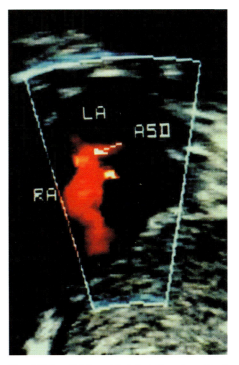

Fig. 1.3.4. Atrial septal defect: Doppler color flow showing the left-to-right shunt through the atrial septal defect (*ASD* atrial septal defect, *LA* left atrium, *RA* right atrium)

transesophageal echocardiography improves the diagnostic accuracy; in uncomplicated cases, surgical decision-making based on echo findings alone.

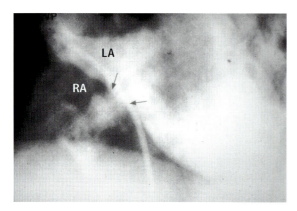

Fig. 1.3.5. Atrial septal defect: angiography showing the contrast medium injected into the left auricular appendage shunting left-to-right through the atrial septal defect (*LA* left atrium, *RA* right atrium, black arrows = upper and lower edge of the atrial septal defect)

▮ **Cardiac catheterization:** in complicated cases and/or in adults with pulmonary hypertension to measure pulmonary vascular resistance and to rule out (or to quantitate the degree of) pulmonary vascular obstructive disease; in selected cases to evaluate the feasibility of closure with interventional cardiology (Fig. 1.3.5).

▮ Indications for surgical treatment

Spontaneous closure of small defects (diameter < 8 mm) occur in a great number of cases. Asymptomatic or mild symptoms: repair at preschool age. Severe symptoms (very rarely): repair in infancy. Adults with pulmonary hypertension: repair in absence of pulmonary vascular obstructive disease. Adults with right-to-left shunt because of other medical problems (pneumonectomy, etc.): repair to treat hypoxemia and to prevent "paradoxical"

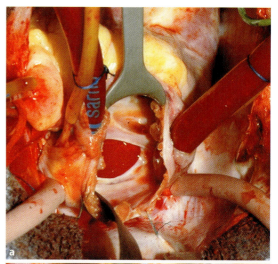

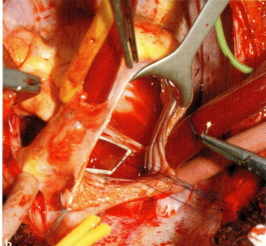

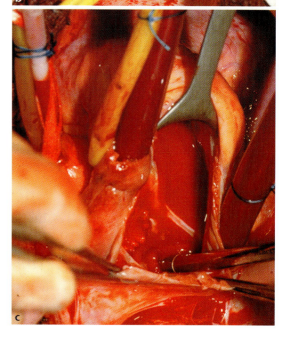

Fig. 1.3.6. Atrial septal defect: patch closure. **a** exposure of the atrial septal defect ostium secundum by retraction of the edges of the right atriotomy, **b** a running suture is used to anastomose a prosthetic patch (in the right lower corner of the photograph) to the rim of the atrial septal defect, **c** prosthetic patch in situ after closure of the atrial septal defect

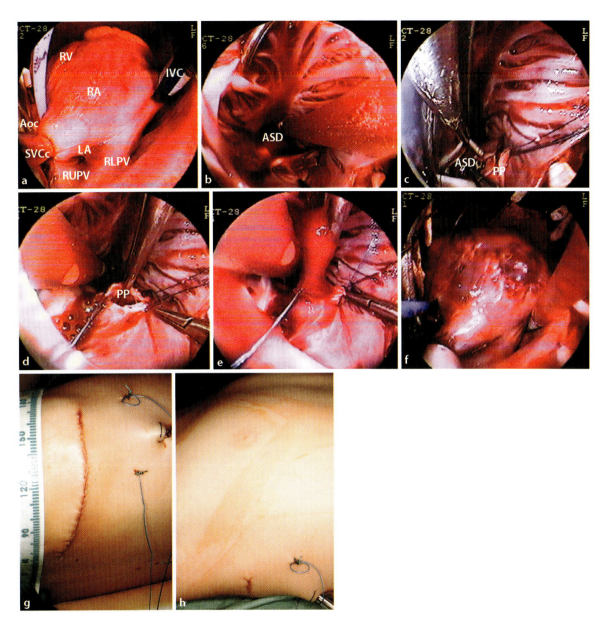

Fig. 1.3.7. Atrial septal defect: surgical approach through postero-lateral right thoracotomy. **a** videoscopic photograph showing the adequate exposure obtained, with aortic cannulation and separate caval veins cannulation (*Aoc* aortic cannula, *IVCc* inferior vena cava cannula, *LA* left atrium, *RA* right atrium, *RLPV* right lower pulmonary vein, *RUPV* right upper pulmonary vein, *RV* right ventricle), **b** adequate exposure of the atrial septal defect through the right atriotomy is shown (*ASD* atrial septal defect), **c** the beginning of the closure of the atrial septal defect with an autologous pericardial patch (*ASD* atrial septal defect, *PP* pericardial patch), **d** the almost completed closure of the atrial septal defect with an autologous pericardial patch (*PP* pericardial patch), **e** videoscopic photograph showing the jet of blood coming from the left atrium at the moment of the air evacuation at the end of the closure of the atrial septal defect, **f** suture closure of the right atriotomy at the end of the procedure, **g** skin wound at the end of the procedure, **h** skin wound at the end of the procedure: anterior and lateral chest wall are completely free from any scar

systemic embolism. Complications of unre-paired atrial septal defect include:

∎ Pulmonary vascular obstructive disease, with subsequent right-to-left shunt at the atrial septal level resulting in cyanosis

∎ Atrial dilation and fibrosis, leading to ar-rhythmias, such as atrial flutter and fibril-lation

∎ Paradoxical embolization, leading to stroke.

∎ Surgical treatment (on cardiopulmonary bypass)

In all cases the defect is approached through a right atriotomy.

∎ *True atrial septal defects*: direct suture or patch closure (Fig. 1.3.6) of the defect (de-pending on the size).

∎ *Sinus venosus*: patch closure of the defect, suturing the patch by leaving the right pulmonary veins on the left side of the patch, with unrestricted communication with the left atrium, and avoiding damage to the sinus node (and the sinus node ar-tery) with the suture line (see chapter "Partial anomalous pulmonary venous connection").

The surgical procedure can be performed through a conventional median sternotomy (Fig. 1.3.6), or through antero-lateral or pos-tero-lateral thoracotomy (Fig. 1.3.7), for a better cosmetic result.

∎ Potential complications

Residual or recurrent atrial septal defect, air embolism (early), systemic and pulmonary thromboembolism (late), supraventricular arrhythmias (particularly in adult patients), pericardial effusion (frequent).

∎ References

Campbell M (1970) Natural history of atrial septal defect. Br Heart J 32:820

Cooley DA, Ellis PR, Bellizi ME (1961) Atrial septal defects of the sinus venosus type: surgical con-siderations. Dis Chest 39:158

Corno AF, Zoia E, Santoro F, Camesasca C, Biagioli B, Grossi A (1992) Epicardial damage induced by topical cooling during pediatric cardiac surgery. Br Heart J 67:174–176

Corno AF, von Segesser LK (1999) Is hypothermia necessary in pediatric cardiac surgery? Eur J Car-diothorac Surg 15:110–111

Corno AF, Chassot PG, Horisberger J, Tozzi P, von Segesser LK (2002) Interatrial communication: mini-invasive surgical approach. Forum Med Suisse 8:40S

Craig RJ, Seltzer A (1968) Natural history and prog-nosis of atrial septal defect. Circulation 37:805–815

Dimic HI, Steinfeld L, Park CC (1973) Symptomatic atrial septal defect in infants. Am Heart J 85:601–604

Ferencz C, Rubin JD, McCarter RJ (1985) Congenital heart disease: prevalence at livebirth. The Balti-more-Washington infant study. Am J Epidemiol 121:31–36

Fyler DC, Buckley LP, Hellenbrand WE, Cohn HE (1980) Report of the New England Regional In-fant Care Program. Pediatrics 65(Suppl):375–461

Galal OM, von Bremen K, Sekarski N, Payot M, Ber-nath MA, Corno AF, Hurni M, von Segesser LK, Fanconi S, Kappenberger L (2001) Cost-compari-son of transcatheter and surgical closure of atrial septal defect in children. Cardiol Young 11(Suppl 1):261

Gibbon JH (1954) Application of a mechanical heart-lung apparatus to cardiac surgery. Minn Med 37:171

Grabitz RG, Joffres MR, Collins-Nakai RL (1988) Congenital heart disease: incidence in the first year of life. The Alberta heritage pediatric cardi-ology program. Am J Epidemiol 128:381–388

Hastreiter AR, Wennemark JT, Miller RA, Paul MH (1962) Secundum atrial septal defects with con-gestive heart failure during infancy and early childhood. Am Heart J 64:467

Haworth SG (1983) Pulmonary vascular disease in secundum atrial septal defect in childhood. Am J Cardiol 51:265–272

Hoffman JIE, Rudolph AM, Danilowicz D (1972) Left to right atrial shunts in infants. Am J Cardiol 30:868–875

Hoffman JIE, Kaplan S (2002) The incidence of con-genital heart disease. J Am Coll Cardiol 39:1890–1900

Lewis FJ, Taufic M (1953) Closure of atrial septal defects with the aid of hypothermia: experimental accomplishments and the report of the one successful case. Surgery 33:52

Marino B, Corno AF, Carotti A, Pasquini L, Giannico S, Guccione P, Bevilacqua M, De Simone G, Marcelletti C (1990) Pediatric cardiac surgery guided by echocardiography. Scand J Thorac Cardiovasc Surg 24:197–201

Phillips SJ, Okies JE, Henken D, Sunderland CO, Starr A (1975) Complex of secundum atrial septal defect and congestive heart failure in infants. J Thorac Cardiovasc Surg 70:696

Sunil GS, Koshy S, Dhinakar S, Shivaprakasha K, Rao SG (2002) Limited right posterior thoracotomy approach to atrial septal defect. Asian Cardiovasc Thorac Ann 10:240–243

Chapter 1.4 Unroofed coronary sinus

Incidence

The unroofed coronary sinus is a very rare malformation.

Morphology

Complete form: the common wall between the coronary sinus and the left atrium (roof of the coronary sinus) is totally absent.

Partial form: an opening is present in the midportion of the wall between the coronary sinus and the left atrium (also called biatrial opening of coronary sinus, or coronary sinus to left atrial fenestration).

Associated anomalies

Persistent left superior vena cava (very frequent), atrial septal defect, common atrium, partial or complete atrioventricular septal defect, mitral stenosis, mitral atresia, tricuspid atresia, tetralogy of Fallot, atrial isomerism.

The persistent superior vena cava usually connects to the left upper corner of the left atrium between the attachment of the left atrial appendage and the left pulmonary veins.

The innominate vein is absent in the great majority of cases, and the right superior vena cava is frequently small or absent.

The inferior vena cava may cross to the left side below the diaphragm and enters the left hemiazygos/vein, which subsequently drains into the left superior vena cava.

The hepatic veins usually enter the inferior aspect of the right atrium, but they too may connect anomalously to the inferior left atrial wall.

Pathophysiology

Right-to-left shunt at atrial level. In the presence of a persistent left superior vena cava, however, cyanosis may be mild or severe depending on the degree of right-to-left shunt.

Diagnosis

■ **Clinical pattern:** increasing cyanosis, polycythemia; cerebral embolism, cerebral abscess.

■ **Electrocardiogram:** atypical.

■ **Chest X-ray:** atypical.

■ **Echocardiogram:** diagnosis can be made by cross sectional and contrast echocardiography or by color flow Doppler; transesophageal echocardiography may improve the diagnostic accuracy (Fig. 1.4.1).

■ **Cardiac catheterization:** suspicion of the diagnosis can be provided by catheter passage or by angiography; angiography may be useful in defining a persistent left superior vena cava (Fig. 1.4.2) and/or inferior vena cava drainage to the left atrium, in addition to defining commonly associated abnormalities.

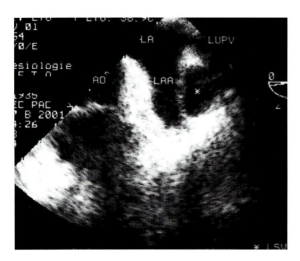

Fig. 1.4.1. Unroofed coronary sinus: echocardiography. Transesophageal view showing the persistence of the left superior vena cava (*AO* aorta, *LA* left atrium, *LAA* left auricular appendage, *LUPV* left upper pulmonary vein, asterisk = persistent left superior vena cava) (photograph courtesy of Dr. Pierre-Guy Chassot)

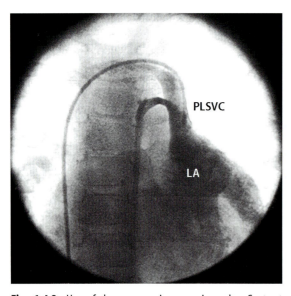

Fig. 1.4.2. Unroofed coronary sinus: angiography. Contrast injection showing the persistent left superior vena cava draining into the left atrium (*LA* left atrium, *PLSVC* persistent left superior vena cava)

■ Indications for surgical treatment

Increasing systemic arterial desaturation, risk of cerebral embolism.

The presence of unroofed coronary sinus has to be taken into consideration in the operative management of the patient undergoing atrial septation or atrio-pulmonary connection.

■ Surgical treatment (on cardiopulmonary bypass)

Simple ligation of the persistent left superior vena cava (without cardiopulmonary bypass) has been reported in the past, in the presence of an innominate vein, but it cannot be recommended because of the risk of potential venous engorgement, facial edema and chylothorax.

Surgical repair can be accomplished with two techniques:

■ complete excision of the entire atrial septum except for a rim of the anterior limbus, in order to preserve the conduction system, followed by suture of a pericardial or synthetic patch as a repositioned atrial septum, leaving all three caval vein orifices on the right side of the patch;

■ rerouting the coronary sinus to the roof of the left atrium, by using the incised atrial septum, and then reconstructing an atrial septum with pericardial or synthetic patch.

Alternative surgical techniques consist of transection of the persistent left superior vena cava and its anastomosis to the right superior vena cava, to the right auricular appendage, or directly to the left pulmonary artery.

▮ Potential complications

Obstruction of the persistent left superior vena cava and/or of the left pulmonary veins, residual or recurrent atrial septal defect, air embolism, supraventricular arrhythmias.

▮ References

Beyens T, Demanet H, Deuvaert FE (1997) Early coronary sinus rerooofing using the left atrial baffle. Ann Thorac Surg 63:832–833

Campbell M, Deuchar DC (1954) The left-sided superior vena cava. Br Heart J 16:423

Chiu IS, Hegerty A, Anderson RH, de Leval MR (1985) The landmarks to the atrioventricular conduction system in hearts with absence or unroofing of the coronary sinus. J Thorac Cardiovasc Surg 90:297

De Leval MR, Ritter DG, McGoon DC, Danielson GK (1975) Anomalous systemic venous connection: surgical considerations. Mayo Clin Proc 50:599

Hahm JK, Park YW, Lee JK, Choi JY, Sul JH, Lee SK, Cho BK, Choe KO (2000) Magnetic resonance imaging of unroofed coronary sinus: three cases. Pediatr Cardiol 21:382–387

Miraldi F, di Gioia CR, Proietti P, de Santis M, d'Amati G, Gallo P (2002) Cardinal vein isomerism: an embryological hypothesis to explain a persistent left superior vena cava draining into the roof of the left atrium in the absence of coronary sinus and atrial septal defect. Cardiovasc Pathol 11:149 152

Nakatani S, Katsuki K, Miyatake K (2002) Images in cardiology: unroofed coronary sinus. Heart 87:278

Quaegebeur J, Kirklin JW, Pacifico AD, Bargeron LM (1979) Surgical experience with unroofed coronary sinus. Ann Thorac Surg 27:418

Raghib G, Ruttenberger HD, Anderson RC, Amplatz K, Adams P, Edwards JE (1965) Termination of the left superior vena cava in left atrium, atrial septal defect, and absence of coronary sinus. A developmental complex. Circulation 31:906–918

Rastelli GC, Ongley PA, Kirklin JW (1965) Surgical correction of common atrium with anomalously connected persistent left superior vena cava: report of a case. Mayo Clin Proc 40:528

Van Son JA, Hambsch J, Mohr FW (1998) Repair of complex unroofed coronary sinus by anastomosis of left to right superior vena cava. Ann Thorac Surg 65:280–281

Vargas-Barron J, Espinola-Zavaleta N, Romero-Cardenas A, Roldan FJ, Keirus C, Hernandez-Reyes P, Miranda-Chavez I, Attie F (2001) Two- and three-dimensional echocardiographic unroofed coronary sinus. J Am Soc Echocardiogr 14:742–744

Watanabe H, Hayashi JI, Sugawara M, Yagi N (1999) Complete unilateral anomalous connection of the left pulmonary veins to the coronary sinus with unroofed coronary sinus syndrome: a case report. Thorac Cardiovasc Surg 47:193–195

CHAPTER 1.5 Atrioventricular septal defect

▮ Incidence

Atrioventricular septal defect is the 4th most common congenital heart defect (7.4% of all congenital heart defects), and the most frequent (50–69%) congenital heart defect in patients with Down syndrome. Atrioventricular septal defect is more frequent in females.

▮ Morphology (Fig. 1.5.1)

Types of atrioventricular septal defect (canal) accordingly with the Rastelli classification:

▮ Type A: the anterior leaflet is divided and attached to the crest of the ventricular septal defect (Fig. 1.5.2).

▮ Type B: the anterior leaflet is divided and chordae from left sided leaflet crosses and inserts into the right ventricle (Fig. 1.5.3).

▮ Type C: the anterior leaflet is ridging (single) with no chordal attachment (free floating) (Fig. 1.5.4).

Types of atrioventricular septal defect accordingly with the Anderson classification:

▮ *Separate atrioventricular orifices, shunting at atrial level*: ostium primum defect, three leaflets left atrioventricular valve (so-called mitral valve with cleft anterior leaflet).

▮ *Separate atrioventricular orifices, shunting at atrial and ventricular levels*: ostium primum defect, space between superior and inferior bridging leaflets of the left atrioventricular valve, inlet ventricular septal defect partially or almost completely

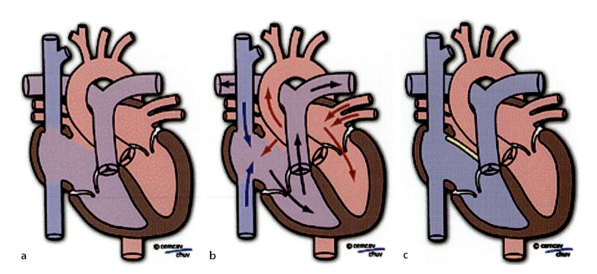

Fig. 1.5.1. Atrioventricular septal defect: ostium primum defect: **a** morphology, **b** pathophysiology, **c** surgery

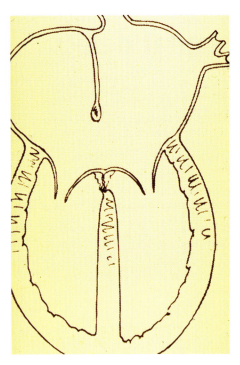

Fig. 1.5.2. Atrioventricular septal defect: morphology. Rastelli classification: type A. The anterior leaflet is divided and attached to the crest of the ventricular septal defect

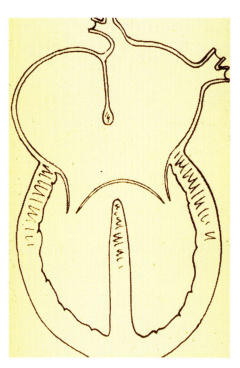

Fig. 1.5.4. Atrioventricular septal defect: morphology. Rastelli classification: type C. The anterior leaflet is ridging (single) with no chordal attachment (free floating)

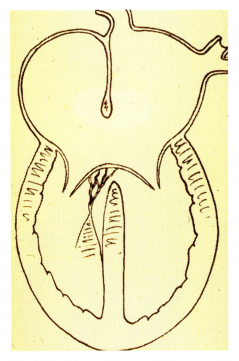

Fig. 1.5.3. Atrioventricular septal defect: morphology. Rastelli classification: type B. The anterior leaflet is divided and chordae from left sided leaflet crosses and inserts in the right ventricle

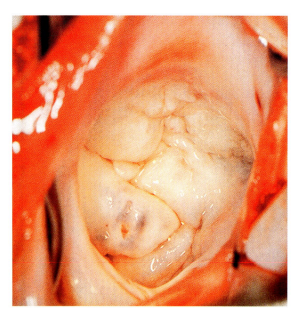

Fig. 1.5.5. Atrioventricular septal defect: morphology of the common atrioventricular valve

closed by fibrous tissue of the atrioventricular valve.

▮ *Common atrioventricular orifice, shunting at atrial and ventricular levels*: ostium primum defect, common atrioventricular valve (Fig. 1.5.5), unrestrictive inlet ventricular septal defect.

▮ Associated anomalies

Patent ductus arteriosus, tetralogy of Fallot or double outlet right ventricle with ventriculo-arterial concordance (more frequent in Down's syndrome), left ventricular outflow tract obstruction (more frequent in patients with separate atrioventricular orifices and those without Down syndrome), unbalanced ventricles (right ventricular dominance more frequent in patients without Down syndrome), persistent left superior vena cava with or without unroofed coronary sinus, additional muscular ventricular septal defects, accessory left atrioventricular valve, single papillary muscle in the left ventricle.

▮ Pathophysiology

Congestive heart failure may appear within the first year of age due to increasing pulmonary blood flow and/or regurgitation of the atrioventricular valve. Infants who tolerate the intracardiac shunt are at risk of developing pulmonary vascular obstructive disease at a young age (less than one year).

Patients with an ostium primum atrioventricular septal defect and no mitral regurgitation present in a manner analogous to those with atrial septal defect.

Patients with atrioventricular septal defect develop elevated pulmonary vascular resistance secondary to right ventricular hypertension, increased pulmonary blood flow and upper airway obstruction, particularly in patients with Down syndrome.

Children with Down syndrome tend to develop pulmonary vascular resistance eleva-

tion earlier than other children, but not necessarily with irreversible lesions.

▮ *Separate atrioventricular orifices, shunting at atrial level*: left-to-right shunt at atrial level, with volume overload of the right heart, increased pulmonary blood flow; left atrioventricular valvular regurgitation of varying degree, from trivial to severe (rarely), with left ventricular volume overload and pulmonary venous congestion in case of severe left atrioventricular valvar regurgitation.

▮ *Separate atrioventricular orifices, shunting at atrial and ventricular levels*: similar to one of the two other forms according to the effective size (restrictive or unrestrictive) of the inlet ventricular septal defect.

▮ *Common atrioventricular orifice, shunting at atrial and ventricular levels*: dependent left-to-right shunt at atrial and ventricular levels, obligatory left-to-right shunt (left ventricle-to-right atrium) in case of moderate to severe left atrioventricular valvular regurgitation, with biventricular volume overload and right ventricular pressure overload, pulmonary hypertension (Fig. 1.5.6).

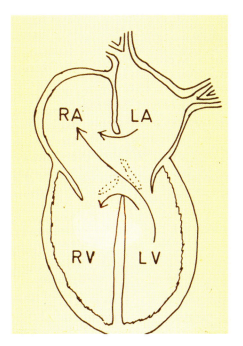

Fig. 1.5.6. Atrioventricular septal defect: pathophysiology

∎ Diagnosis

On examination there is a holosystolic murmur at the left lower sternal border and apex; in addition, the second sound is accentuated, with a third sound.

∎ Clinical pattern:
- separate atrioventricular orifices, shunting at atrial level (more frequent in patients without Down syndrome): asymptomatic or with mild symptoms of congestive heart failure and/or upper respiratory infections;
- separate atrioventricular orifices, shunting at atrial and ventricular levels: concomitant with the pathophysiology;
- common atrioventricular orifice, shunting at atrial and ventricular levels (more frequent in Down syndrome): symptoms from the first months of life because of congestive heart failure, poor physical growth, recurrent respiratory infections and pulmonary hypertension; early development of pulmonary vascular obstructive disease (especially in Down syndrome).

∎ Electrocardiogram: prolonged PR interval, counterclockwise direction of the QRS axis, with or without right ventricular or biventricular hypertrophy.

∎ Chest X-ray:
- separate atrioventricular orifices: enlargement of the morphologically right chambers;
- common atrioventricular orifice: enlargement of all four chambers, increased pulmonary vascularity.

∎ Echocardiogram: diagnostic in all cases for the cardiac morphology (Figs. 1.5.7 and 1.5.8); in uncomplicated cases, surgical decision-making based on echocardiography.

∎ Cardiac catheterization: evidence of the "cleft" of the left atrioventricular valve (Fig. 1.5.9) or the "goose neck" deformity of the

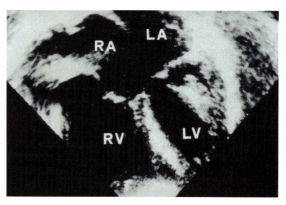

Fig. 1.5.7. Atrioventricular septal defect ostium primum: echocardiography. Four chamber view showing the ostium primum atrioventricular septal defect, the atrioventricular leaflets inserted at the same level and the absence of the ventricular component of the defect (*LA* left atrium, *LV* left ventricle, *RA* right atrium, *RV* right ventricle) (reproduced with permission from Marino B, Thiene G (1990) Atlante di anatomia ecocardiografica delle cardiopatie congenite, USES, Firenze)

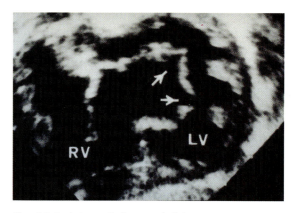

Fig. 1.5.8. Atrioventricular septal defect common atrioventricular orifice: echocardiography. Short axis view showing the common atrioventricular orifice (arrows) with insertion on both ventricles (*LV* left ventricle, *RV* right ventricle) (reproduced with permission from Marino B, Thiene G (1990) Atlante di anatomia ecocardiografica delle cardiopatie congenite, USES, Firenze)

left ventricular outflow tract (Fig. 1.5.10) because of the inlet-outlet septal disproportion and the abnormal location of the left ventricular outflow tract;

cardiac catheterization is necessary in:
- patients with separate atrioventricular orifices in presence of severe symptoms in infancy;

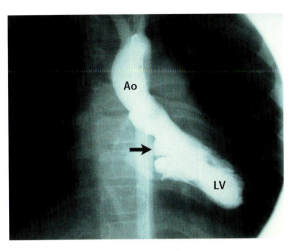

Fig. 1.5.9. Atrioventricular septal defect ostium primum: angiography (*Ao* aorta, *LV* left ventricle, *arrow* "cleft" of the left atrioventricular valve)

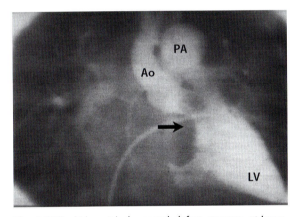

Fig. 1.5.10. Atrioventricular septal defect common atrioventricular orifice: angiography (*Ao* aorta, *LV* left ventricle, *PA* pulmonary artery, *arrow* "goose neck" deformity of the left ventricular outflow tract)

– patients with common atrioventricular orifices after 6–8 months of age to measure pulmonary vascular resistance and to rule out (or to quantitate the degree of) pulmonary vascular obstructive disease;
– patients with complex malformation.

■ Indications for surgical treatment

■ *Separate atrioventricular orifices, shunting at the atrial level:*
– asymptomatic or mild symptoms: repair at preschool age,

– severe symptoms: repair in infancy.
■ *Separate atrioventricular orifices, shunting at atrial and ventricular levels:*
restrictive ventricular septal defect: as for those with separate orifices,
– unrestrictive ventricular septal defect: as for those with common orifice.
■ *Common atrioventricular orifice, shunting at atrial and ventricular levels:*
– repair within 4–6 months of age (before the development of pulmonary vascular obstructive disease).
■ *Complex atrioventricular septal defect:*
– associated anomalies: palliation (shunt, pulmonary artery banding, other),
– unbalanced ventricles: pulmonary artery banding, univentricular repair, heart transplant.

■ Surgical treatment (on cardiopulmonary bypass)

In all cases the surgical approach is from a right atriotomy. In the case of the double patch technique, a prosthetic patch (PTFE, Dacron, Teflon) is used for the ventricular component, and a biological patch (autologous or heterologous pericardium) for the atrial component. In the case of the single patch technique, either a prosthetic or biological patch is used accordingly with the surgical preferences.

■ *Separate atrioventricular orifices, shunting at the atrial level:* patch closure of ostium primum +/– suture of the space between the bridging leaflets ("cleft") (Fig. 1.5.11).
■ *Separate atrioventricular orifices, shunting at the atrial and ventricular levels:* as above with patch closure of the ventricular septal defect.
■ *Common atrioventricular orifice, shunting at the atrial and ventricular levels:*
– single patch closure of atrial and ventricular septal defects, division of the bridging leaflets and resuspension to the patch, with or without suture of the so-called "cleft"

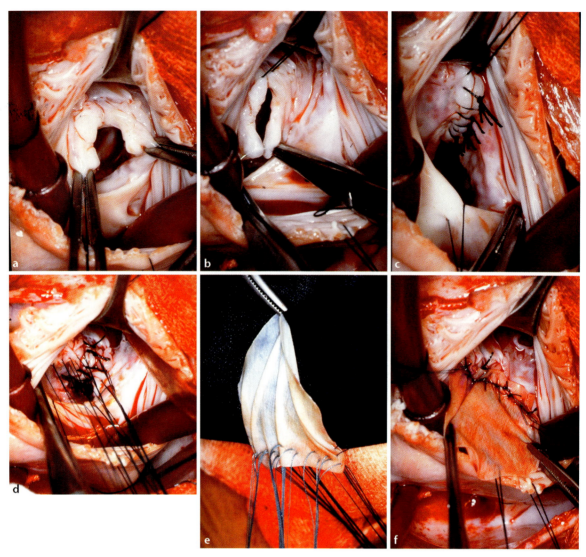

Fig. 1.5.11. Atrioventricular septal defect: separate atrioventricular orifices, shunting at the atrial level. Surgical repair: **a** exposure of the intracardiac anatomy by retraction of the edges of the right atriotomy; identification (with two forceps) of the space between the bridging leaflets or "cleft" of the left atrioventricular valve, **b** with traction on the interrupted suture in correspondence of the annulus of the atrioventricular valve, placement of the first of the interrupted sutures used to close the "cleft", **c** complete closure of the "cleft" with interrupted sutures, **d** interrupted sutures in correspon-dence of the annulus to separate the right from the left atrioventricular valve with the lower portion of the patch closing the ostium primum defect, **e** the other side of the interrupted sutures in correspondence of the heterologous pericardial patch used to close the ostium primum defect, **f** the interrupted sutures ligated to place the lower portion of the heterologous pericardial patch used to close the ostium primum defect in correspondence of the atrioventricular annulus

– or:
double patch closure of atrial and ventricular septal defects (Fig. 1.5.12), bridging leaflets, "sandwiched" between atrial and ventricular patches, with or without suture of the so-called "cleft"

in both techniques: test of the competence of the left atrioventricular valve with injection of saline solution under pressure in the left ventricle; in case of significant regurgitation, adjustment of the repair by shifting the valvular leaflets with additional sutures; caution

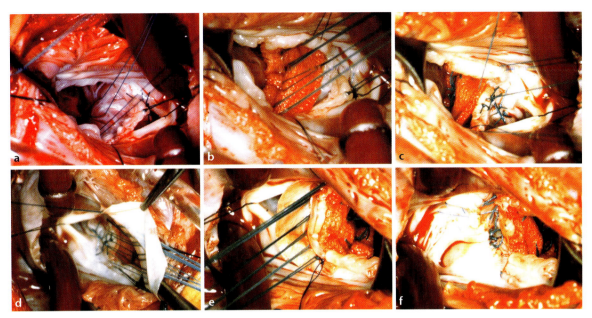

Fig. 1.5.12. Atrioventricular septal defect: common atrioventricular orifice, shunting at the atrial and ventricular levels. Surgical repair: **a** after exposure of the intracardiac anatomy by retraction of the edges of the right atriotomy and closure by interrupted sutures of the "cleft" (see Fig. 1.5.11), placement of interrupted sutures on the upper rim of the interventricular septum, **b** attachment of the prosthetic patch to the upper rim of the interventricular septum to close the ventricular component of the defect, **c** attachment of the upper portion of the prosthetic patch closing the ventricular component of the defect to the tissue of the bridging leaflet (with the "cleft" previously closed), **d** attachment of the interrupted sutures, previously utilized to fix the upper portion of the prosthetic patch to the bridging leaflet, to the lower portion of the pericardial patch that will be utilized to close the atrial component of the defect, **e** bridging leaflet sandwiched between ventricular (prosthetic) and atrial (pericardial) patch, **f** pericardial patch in situ, ready to complete the closure of the atrial component of the defect

to avoid creation of left atrioventricular valvular stenosis or subvalvular aortic stenosis.

■ Potential complications

Residual or recurrent atrial and/or ventricular septal defect, complete atrioventricular block, left atrioventricular valvar regurgitation and/or stenosis, left ventricular outflow tract obstruction, pulmonary arterial hypertensive crisis.

■ References

Aimé E, Frigiola A, Rovida M, Corno AF, De Ambroggi L (1993) Endomyocardial permanent pace-maker implantation in infants and children with postoperative a-v block. PACE 16:1143

Ando M, Fraser CD (2001) Prosthetic mitral valve replacement after atrioventricular septal defect repair: a technique for small children. Ann Thorac Surg 72:907–909

Becker AE, Anderson RH (1982) Atrioventricular septal defect: what's in a name? J Thorac Cardiovasc Surg 83:461–469

Ben-Shachar G, Moller JH, Castaneda-Zuniga W, Edwards JE (1981) Signs of membranous subaortic stenosis appearing after correction of persistent common atrioventricular canal. Am J Cardiol 48:340–344

Berger TJ, Blackstone EH, Kirklin JW, Bargeron LM, Hazelrig JB, Turner ME (1979) Survival and probability of cure without and with operation in complete atrioventricular canal. Ann Thorac Surg 27:104–111

Bharati S, Lev M (1973) The spectrum of common atrioventricular orifice (canal). Am Heart J 86:553–561

Corno AF, Marino B, Catena G, Marcelletti C (1988) Atrioventricular septal defects with severe left ventricular hypoplasia. Staged palliation. J Thorac Cardiovasc Surg 96:249–252

Corno AF, Carta MG, Giannico S (1989) Pulmonary artery banding through median sternotomy. Cl Res 37:91A

Corno AF, Zoia E, Santoro F, Camesasca C, Biagioli B, Grossi A (1992) Epicardial damage induced by topical cooling during pediatric cardiac surgery. Br Heart J 67:174–176

Corno AF (1995) Congenital septal defects: role of the pulmonary artery banding on 1995. In: D'Alessandro LC (ed) Heart Surgery 1995. CESI, Rome, pp 167–175

Corno AF, von Segesser LK (1999) Is hypothermia necessary in pediatric cardiac surgery? Eur J Cardiothorac Surg 15:110–111

Corno AF (2000) Surgery for congenital heart disease. Curr Opinion Cardiol 15:238–243

Corno AF, Sekarski N, von Segesser LK (2002) Remote control of pulmonary blood flow: a dream comes true. Swiss Med Weekly 132:423–424

Crawford FA, Stroud MR (2001) Surgical repair of complete atrioventricular septal defect. Ann Thorac Surg 72:1621–1628

De Biase L, Di Ciommo V, Ballerini L, Bevilacqua M, Marcelletti C, Marino B (1986) Prevalence of left-sided obstructive lesions in patients with atrioventricular canal without Down's syndrome. J Thorac Cardiovasc Surg 91:467

Digilio MC, Marino B, Cicini MP, Gianotti A, Corno AF, Dallapiccola B (1991) Ricorrenza di cardiopatie congenite in famiglia di pazienti con canale atrioventricolare senza anomalie cromosomiche. G Ital Cardiol 21(Suppl II):29

Ebels T, Anderson RH, Devine WA, Debich DE, Penkoske PA, Zuberbuhler JR (1990) Anomalies of the left atrioventricular valve and related ventricular septal morphology in atrioventricular septal defects. J Thorac Cardiovasc Surg 99:299–307

Ebert PA, Goor DA (1978) Complete atrioventricular canal malformations: further clarification of the anatomy of the common leaflet and its relationship to the VSD in surgical correction. Ann Thorac Surg 25:134–143

Epstein ML, Moller JH, Amplatz K, Nicoloff DM (1979) Pulmonary artery banding in infants with complete atrioventricular canal. J Thorac Cardiovasc Surg 78:28

Ferencz C, Rubin JD, McCarter RJ (1985) Congenital heart disease: prevalence at livebirth. The Baltimore-Washington infant study. Am J Epidemiol 121:31–36

Frescura C, Thiene G, Franceschini E, Talenti E, Mazzucco A (1987) Pulmonary vascular disease in infants with complete atrioventricular septal defect. Int J Cardiol 15:91

Fyler DC, Buckley LP, Hellenbrand WE, Cohn HE (1980) Report of the New England Regional Infant Care Program. Pediatrics 65(Suppl):375–461

Giamberti A, Marino B, Guccione P, Pasquini L, Iorio F, Corno AF, De Simone G, Marcelletti C (1990) Correzione chirurgica del canale atrioventricolare senza cateterismo cardiaco. G Ital Cardiol 20:144–147

Hoffman JIE, Kaplan S (2002) The incidence of congenital heart disease. J Am Coll Cardiol 39:1890–1900

Kirklin JW, Blackstone EH (1979) Management of the infant with complete atrioventricular canal. J Thorac Cardiovasc Surg 78:32

Marino B, Iorio F, Corno AF, Pierli C, Annichiarico M, Giamberti A, Papa M, Marcelletti C (1988) Correzione chirurgica del canale atrioventricolare senza cateterismo cardiaco. Criteri per la selezione dei pazenti. Cardiol 33(Suppl II):19

Marino B, Guccione P, Corno AF, Papa M, Marcelletti C, Dallapiccola B (1989) Facial anomalies in patients with atrioventricular canal and normal chromosomes: the non-Down atrioventricular canal. Eur Heart J 10:285

Marino B, Guccione P, Corno AF, Marcelletti C, Dallapiccola B (1989) Atrioventricular canal, normal chromosomes and phenotypic anomalies. Cl Res 37:97A

Marino B, Corno AF (1989) Parental transmission of congenital heart diseases. Am J Cardiol 63:262

Marino B, Corno AF, Carotti A, Pasquini L, Giannico S, Guccione P, Bevilacqua M, De Simone G, Marcelletti C (1990) Pediatric cardiac surgery guided by echocardiography. Scand J Thorac Cardiovasc Surg 24:197–201

Marino B, Vairo U, Corno AF, Nava S, Guccione P, Calabrò R, Marcelletti C (1990) Atrioventricular canal in Down syndrome. Am J Dis Child 144:1120–1122

Rastelli GC, Kirklin JW, Titus JL (1966) Anatomic observations of complete form of persistent common atrioventricular canal. With special reference to atrioventricular valves. Mayo Clin Proc 41:296–308

Rastelli GC, Ongley PA, Kirklin JW, McGoon DC (1968) Surgical repair of complete form of persistent common atrioventricular canal. J Thorac Cardiovasc Surg 55:299

Studer M, Blackstone EH, Kirklin JW, Pacifico AD, Soto B, Chung GKT, Kirklin JK, Bargeron LM (1982) Determinants of early and late results of repair of atrioventricular septal (canal) defects. J Thorac Cardiovasc Surg 84:523

Suzuki T, Fukuda T (2002) Two-patch repair of complete atrioventricular septal defect using a small ventricular patch. Ann Thorac Surg 74:1718–1719

Weintraub RG, Brawn WJ, Venables AW, Mee RBB (1990) Two-patch repair of complete atrioventricular septal defect in the first year of life. J Thorac Cardiovasc Surg 99:320

I Incidence

The ventricular septal defect is the most common congenital heart disease at one week of age and throughout the first three decades of life: 32.1% of all patients with congenital heart disease have ventricular septal defects, 0.3–0.5/1000 live births have significant ventricular septal defects requiring management. Premature infants have a much higher incidence: ten times as high as full term babies. Ventricular septal defect is most frequent in females.

I Morphology (Figs. 1.6.1 and 1.6.2)

I *Perimembranous ventricular septal defect* (Fig. 1.6.3): the membranous septum is very small, therefore ventricular septal defects usually extend into the surrounding muscle septum, and this is called perimembranous ventricular septal defect; this type of ventricular septal defect is the most common after infancy, accounting for 75% of all ventricular septal defects; defect surrounding the membranous septum, at the meeting point of the three right ventricular components (inlet, apical trabecular and outlet); diagnostic feature is a fibrous continuity between the leaflets of the aortic and tricuspid valve; can extend to open mostly to inlet or outlet of the right ventricle, or can be confluent;

juxtacrux ventricular septal defect: particular perimembranous defect associated with straddling and overriding of the tricuspid valve; diagnostic feature is malalignment between the atrial and ventricular septum.

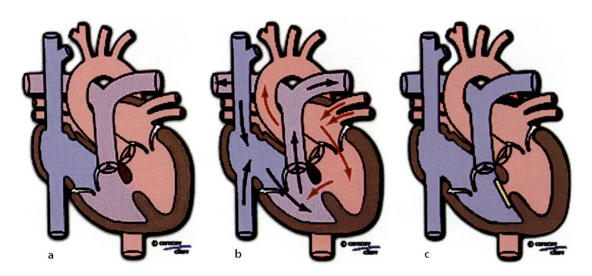

Fig. 1.6.1. Ventricular septal defect: **a** morphology, **b** pathophysiology, **c** surgery

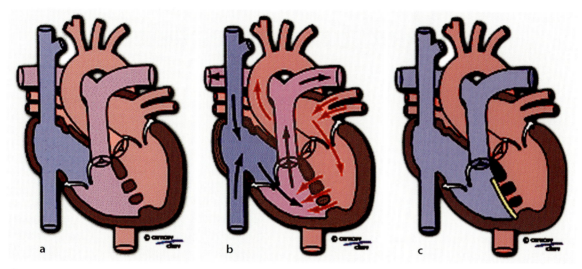

Fig. 1.6.2. Multiple ventricular septal defects: **a** morphology, **b** pathophysiology, **c** surgery

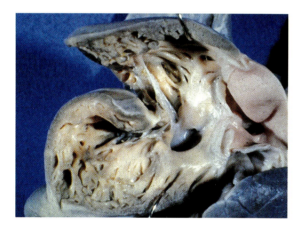

Fig. 1.6.3. Ventricular septal defect. Morphology of perimembranous ventricular septal defect (photograph courtesy of Dr. Bruno Marino)

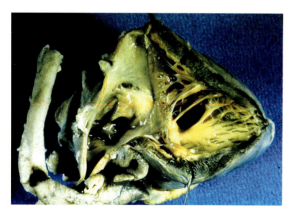

Fig. 1.6.4. Ventricular septal defect. Morphology of muscular ventricular septal defect (photograph courtesy of Dr. Bruno Marino)

■ *Muscular ventricular septal defect* (Fig. 1.6.4): this is the second most common type of ventricular septal defect after infancy; in infancy, muscular ventricular septal defect is the most frequent type, but most of them, very small in size, undergo complete spontaneous closure; a defect which has completely muscular rims; can be situated anywhere within the septum, but can be subdivided into those opening to the inlet, trabecular or outlet components of the right ventricle.

■ *Doubly committed juxta-arterial ventricular septal defect:* defect limited superiorly by fibrous continuity between the leaflets of the pulmonary and aortic valves, because of absence of the outlet septum and the septal component of the subpulmonary infundibulum; can have a muscular posterior rim, which protects axis for atrioventricular conduction, or can extend to become perimembranous.

■ *Multiple ventricular septal defects:* combination of multiple muscular defects or of one or more muscular defect(s) co-existing with perimembranous or juxta-arterial defects.

■ *Inlet ventricular septal defects:* see chapter "Atrioventricular septal defects".

▌ Relation to the conduction axis

Importance of morphologic classification is that it provides a guide to the conduction axis. The conduction axis is always postero-inferior to the perimembranous defect (to the surgeon's right hand when working through the right atrium), except when there is overriding of the tricuspid valve (juxta-crux defect). The conduction axis is antero-superior to the muscular inlet defect and relatively distant from other muscular defects.

The postero-inferior muscle bar protects the axis in a doubly committed defect which is not perimembranous.

▌ Associated anomalies

A ventricular septal defect may coexist with nearly all varieties of congenital heart disease, but the interventricular communication is only considered the primary lesion when the left-to-right shunt at the ventricular level is the dominant hemodynamic lesion.

Atrial septal defect, partial (or total) anomalous pulmonary venous connection, infundibular or pulmonary valvular stenosis, double-chambered right ventricle, mitral stenosis, discrete (fibrous) subvalvar aortic stenosis, aortic valvular regurgitation (Laubry-Pezzi syndrome), aneurysm of the sinuses of Valsalva (right coronary sinus is the most common), patent ductus arteriosus, aortic coarctation, aortic arch hypoplasia or interruption are the most common lesions which complicate the ventricular septal defect seen as the primary lesion.

▌ Pathophysiology

The larger the ventricular septal defect, the more the left ventricular pressure is transmitted to the right ventricle. When the ventricular septal defect is more than 50% of the area of the aortic root (unrestrictive defect), the right ventricular pressure equalizes with the left ventricular pressure. The deter-

mining factor for the amount of left-to-right shunting at that point becomes the ratio between systemic and pulmonary vascular resistance.

- ▌ *Small (restrictive) ventricular septal defect:* little left-to-right shunt, normal right ventricular pressure, without enlargement of the left atrium and left ventricle.
- ▌ *Moderate ventricular septal defect:* consistent left-to-right shunt, mild pulmonary hypertension; after 2–3 years of age, possibility of left atrial enlargement, signs of left ventricular volume overload.
- ▌ *Large ventricular septal defect:* important left-to-right shunt, severe pulmonary hypertension (systemic level); left atrial enlargement, left ventricular volume overload.
- ▌ *Ventricular septal defect with aortic regurgitation:* pathophysiology depending on the size of the ventricular septal defect and on the entity of the aortic regurgitation; the latter may cause volume overload of the left ventricle and/or of the right ventricle.
- ▌ *Multiple ventricular septal defects:* pathophysiology depending on the size, number and location of the defects.
- ▌ *Ventricular septal defect with aortic coarctation:* see chapter "Aortic coarctation".
- ▌ *Ventricular septal defect with aortic arch interruption* (see chapter "Aortic arch interruption").

▌ Diagnosis

The murmur of the ventricular septal defect is due to left-to-right shunting at the ventricular level. Small ventricular septal defects are typically louder than larger ones. The murmur of a ventricular septal defect is heard best at the left lower sternal border. A loud third heart sound or diastolic rumble is heard with large left-to-right shunting due to increased flow across the mitral valve. A thrill is felt in many cases, particularly beyond infancy.

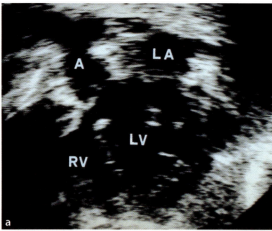

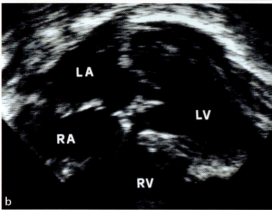

Fig. 1.6.5. Ventricular septal defect: echocardiography. **a** short axis view showing a subaortic perimembranous ventricular septal defect, **b** 4-chamber view showing a perimembranous ventricular septal defect (*A* aorta, *LA* left atrium, *LV* left ventricle, *RA* right atrium, *RV* right ventricle) (reproduced with permission from Marino B, Thiene G (1990) Atlante di anatomia ecocardiografica delle cardiopatie congenite, USES, Firenze)

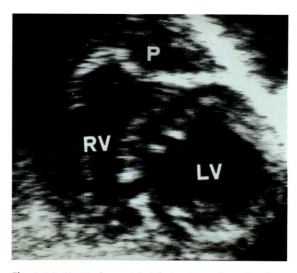

Fig. 1.6.6. Ventricular septal defect: echocardiography. Short axis view showing a muscular ventricular septal defect (*LV* left ventricle, *P* pulmonary artery, *RV* right ventricle) (reproduced with permission from Marino B, Thiene G (1990) Atlante di anatomia ecocardiografica delle cardiopatie congenite, USES, Firenze)

Right-to-left shunting at the level of the ventricular septal defect is not audible due to the small pressure difference between the right and left ventricles.

▪ **Clinical pattern:**
- small (restrictive) ventricular septal defect: asymptomatic;
- moderate ventricular septal defect: usually asymptomatic, rarely congestive heart failure and/or recurrent upper respiratory infections;
- large ventricular septal defect: generally congestive heart failure after 2–3 months of age, failure to growth, recurrent pulmonary infections.

▪ **Electrocardiogram:**
- small (restrictive) ventricular septal defect: normal;
- moderate ventricular septal defect: left ventricular dilatation;
- large ventricular septal defect: biventricular hypertrophy, left atrial and left ventricular dilatation.

▪ **Chest X-ray:**
- small (restrictive) ventricular septal defect: normal;
- moderate ventricular septal defect: mild cardiomegaly (left ventricular enlargement), increased pulmonary vascularity;
- large ventricular septal defect: severe cardiomegaly (left and right ventricular enlargement), pulmonary congestion.

▪ **Echocardiogram:** diagnostic in all cases by recognition of the cardiac morphology and the associated lesions; in uncomplicated cases, surgical decision-making based on echo findings alone;

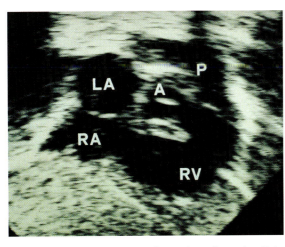

Fig. 1.6.7. Ventricular septal defect: echocardiography. Right oblique view showing a doubly committed juxta-arterial ventricular septal defect (*A* aorta, *LA* left atrium, *P* pulmonary artery, *RA* right atrium, *RV* right ventricle)

– perimembranous ventricular septal defect: seen from precordial or subcostal view that images the area just below the aortic root (Fig. 1.6.5);
– muscular ventricular septal defect (Fig. 1.6.6): better seen with Doppler color flow;
– doubly committed juxta-arterial ventricular septal defect: subcostal or precordial view (Fig. 1.6.7), with Doppler color flow; transesophageal echocardiography provides better definition of morphological and functional details (Fig. 1.6.8).

■ **Cardiac catheterization:** in patients with moderate ventricular septal defect, necessary to quantitate the left-to-right shunt; in patients with large ventricular septal defect, necessary to quantitate the degree of pulmonary

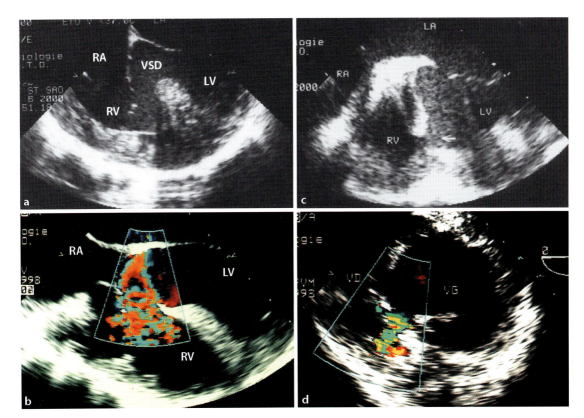

Fig. 1.6.8. Ventricular septal defect: echocardiography. **a** transesophageal view showing a perimembranous ventricular septal defect (*LV* left ventricle, *RA* right atrium, *RV* right ventricle, *VSD* ventricular septal defect) (photograph courtesy of Dr. Pierre Guy-Chassot), **b** transesophageal color Doppler with the left-to-right shunt through the perimembranous ventricular septal defect (photograph courtesy of Dr. Pierre Guy-Chassot), **c** transesophageal view showing a muscular ventricular septal defect (*LA* left atrium, white arrow = muscular ventricular septal defect) (photograph courtesy of Dr. Pierre Guy-Chassot), **d** transesophageal color Doppler with the left-to-right shunt through the muscular ventricular septal defect (photograph courtesy of Dr. Pierre Guy-Chassot)

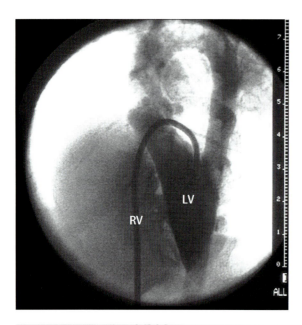

Fig. 1.6.9. Ventricular septal defect: angiography. Left ventricular injection showing multiple ventricular septal defects (*LV* left ventricle, *RV* right ventricle)

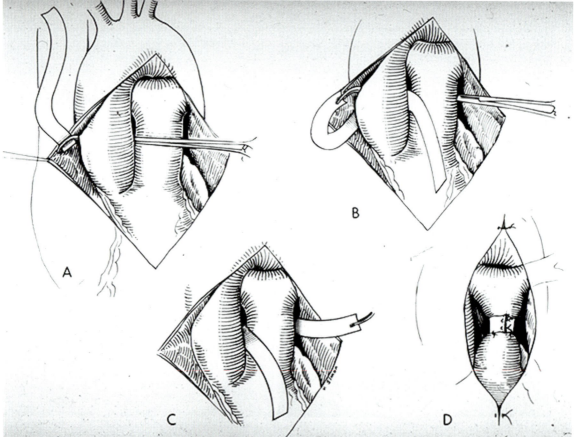

Fig. 1.6.10. Ventricular septal defect: surgery. Pulmonary artery banding: schematic drawing of the palliative procedure through a median sternotomy, with a surgical instrument encircling the ascending aorta with the band (**A**), the same surgical instrument grabbing the other end of the band after having encircled ascending aorta and pulmonary artery (**B**), with the exclusion maneuver the band remaining around the pulmonary artery only (**C**) and the band fixed with sutures around the main pulmonary artery to reduce the distal pulmonary artery flow and pressures (**D**)

hypertension and pulmonary vascular resistance; left ventricular cineangiography necessary to define precisely the location and number of multiple ventricular septal defects (Fig. 1.6.9); in selected cases of muscular defects to evaluate the feasibility of closure with interventional catheterization. The best views to visualize the ventricular septal defect on a left ventricular angiogram are as follows:

- perimembranous, mid muscular and apical ventricular septal defects are best seen in the left anterior oblique views,
- anterior muscular and subpulmonary ventricular septal defects are best seen in the right anterior oblique views,
- posterior muscular and inlet ventricular septal defects are best seen in the hepatoclavicular (40° left anterior oblique and 40° cranial angulation).

∎ Indications for surgical treatment

∎ *Spontaneous diminution in size:*
- Perimembranous ventricular septal defects have a tendency to become smaller (about 50% of them do so); therefore, it is worthwhile allowing the child to grow since these ventricular septal defects may close spontaneously; spontaneous closure of defects in most instances involves tricuspid valve tissue.
- Muscular ventricular septal defects typically become smaller and may close spontaneously.
- Doubly committed juxta-arterial ventricular septal defects are typically large and do not become smaller spontaneously.
∎ *Development of pulmonary vascular obstructive disease:* Rarely encountered nowadays; it can occur after one or two years of age. Surgery is contraindicated if any of the following are present:
  - Pulmonary vascular resistance higher than 8–10 Wood units.
  - Pulmonary vascular resistance not responsive to pulmonary vasodilators such as oxygen or nitrous oxide.

- Predominantly right-to-left shunting across the ventricular septal defect.
∎ *Indication for surgery:*
  Small (restrictive) ventricular septal defect: no indication for surgery, in the absence of aortic regurgitation; prevention of bacterial endocarditis.
- Moderate ventricular septal defect: surgical treatment (defect closure) usually after the first or second year of age.
- Large ventricular septal defect: surgical treatment (defect closure) usually within 6 months of age.
- Ventricular septal defect with aortic regurgitation: in the presence of ventricular septal defect even of small size, indication for surgery (defect closure with or without aortic valve plasty) at the first appearance of (or at worsening of a previously seen) aortic regurgitation.

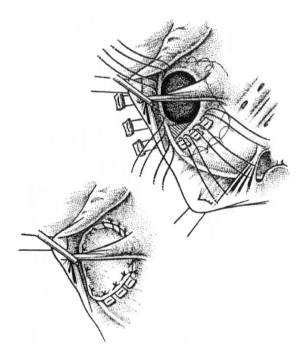

Fig. 1.6.11. Ventricular septal defect: surgery. Patch closure of the defect from a right atriotomy, with retraction of the tricuspid valve (reproduced with permission from Merrick AF, Lal M, Anderson RH, Shore DF (1999) Management of ventricular septal defect: a survey of practice in the United Kingdom. Ann Thorac Surg 68:983–988)

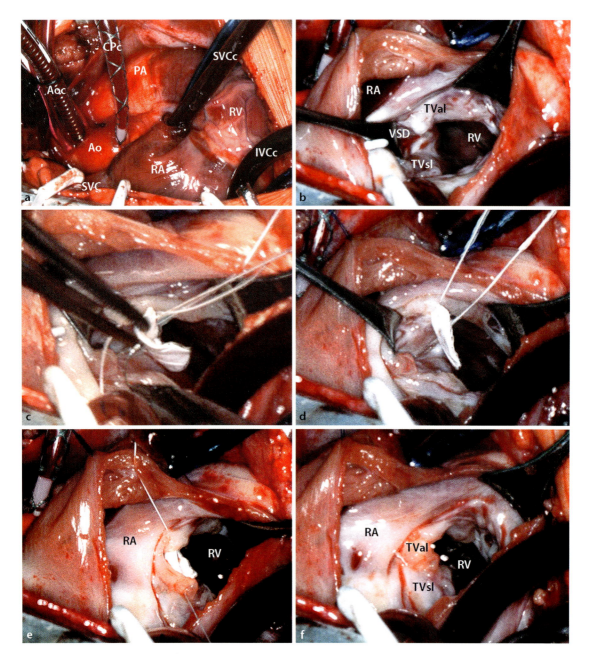

Fig. 1.6.12. Ventricular septal defect: surgery. Patch closure of the defect from a right atriotomy: **a** preparation for the cardiopulmonary bypass (*Ao* aorta, *Aoc* aortic cannula (inserted into the ascending aorta), *CPc* cannula for cardioplegia (inserted into the aortic root), *IVCc* cannula for the inferior vena cava, *PA* pulmonary artery, *RA* right atrium, *RV* right ventricle, *SVC* superior vena cava, *SVCc* cannula for the superior vena cava (inserted from the right atrium), **b** after oblique right atriotomy, exposure of the perimembranous ventricular septal defect by retracting the anterior and the septal leaflet of the tricuspid valve (*TVal* tricuspid valve, anterior leaflet, *TVsl* tricuspid valve, septal leaflet, *VSD* ven- tricular septal defect), **c** the first stitches of the running su- ture are used to fix the PTFE patch to the inferior rim of the ventricular septal defect, **d** the PTFE patch is now fixed to the inferior rim of the ventricular septal defect, **e** the two running sutures on both sides of the defect are almost com- pleted, and the PTFE patch is now almost completely fixed, with the exception of the superior rim of the ventricular sep- tal defect, **f** after completion of the patch closure of ventric- ular septal defect and relief of the traction on the leaflets of the tricuspid valve, the PTFE patch is not visible any more from the right atrium

▮ *Palliative treatment (pulmonary artery banding, Fig. 1.6.10)* has to be considered in the following cases:
  - Multiple defects under 6 months of age, especially when requiring ventriculotomy for repair;
  - Association with aortic coarctation or aortic arch interruption;
  - Association with other congenital non-cardiac anomalies (omphalocele, esophageal atresia, diaphragmatic hernia);
  - Severely undernourished babies;
  - Active respiratory infections, uncontrollable because of severe heart failure, precluding cardiopulmonary bypass.

▮ Surgical treatment (on cardiopulmonary bypass)

The defect is generally closed with a patch (PTFE, Dacron, Teflon accordingly with the surgical preferences; very rarely is pericardium used), sutured with running sutures (rarely with interrupted sutures). Direct closure with Teflon pledgets is used only for very small defects.

▮ *Perimembranous ventricular septal defect:* patch closure of the defect through a right atriotomy and tricuspid valve retraction (Figs. 1.6.11 and 1.6.12) or disinsertion; patch closure through right ventriculotomy (Figs. 1.6.13 and 1.6.14) in case of associated infundibular obstruction requiring right ventriculotomy for relief.
▮ *Muscular ventricular septal defect:* patch closure of the defect through a right atriotomy and tricuspid valve retraction; more rarely through a right ventriculotomy; very rarely through an apical left ventriculotomy.
▮ *Doubly committed juxta-arterial ventricular septal defect:* patch closure of the defect through a right atriotomy and tricuspid retraction or through an aortotomy or through an incision of the main pulmonary artery, accordingly with the position of the defect and its relationship with the semilu-

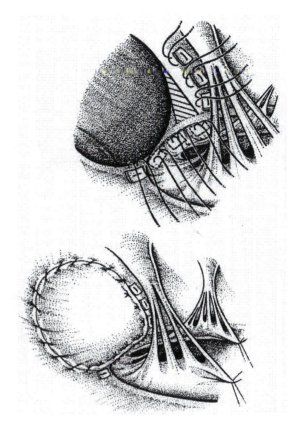

Fig. 1.6.13. Ventricular septal defect: surgery. Patch closure of the defect from a right ventriculotomy (reproduced with permission from Merrick AF, Lal M, Anderson RH, Shore DF (1999) Management of ventricular septal defect: a survey of practice in the United Kingdom. Ann Thorac Surg 68:983–988)

nar valves, with the need of treatment of prolapsed aortic leaflet or of a right ventricular outflow tract enlargement, and with the size of the ascending aorta.
▮ *Multiple ventricular septal defects:* multiple or large single patch closure of the defects through a right atriotomy (Fig. 1.6.15); more rarely through a right ventriculotomy; very rarely through an apical left ventriculotomy.

▮ Potential complications

Residual or recurrent ventricular septal defect, complete atrioventricular block, pulmonary arterial hypertensive crisis.

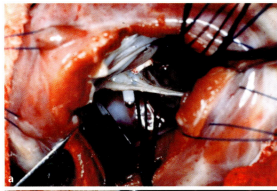

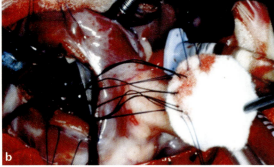

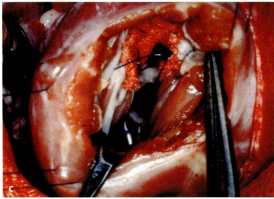

Fig. 1.6.14. Ventricular septal defect: patch closure from right ventriculotomy. **a** exposure of the ventricular septal defect from a right ventriculotomy, with 3 interrupted pledgeted sutures anchored to the septal leaflet of the tricuspid valve, **b** the 3 interrupted pledgeted sutures anchored to the septal leaflet of the tricuspid valve have been anastomosed to the inferior rim of the prosthetic patch, as well as the beginning of the 2 running sutures to be utilized to anastomose the patch to the rest of the defect, **c** the 3 interrupted pledgeted sutures have been tied to the septal leaflet of the tricuspid valve, and the 2 running sutures completed the patch closure of the rest of the defect

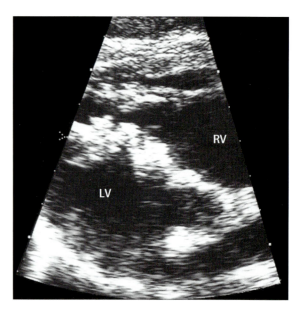

Fig. 1.6.15. Ventricular septal defect: post-operative echocardiography. Multiple ventricular septal defects (same patient as in Fig. 1.6.8) after surgical repair (*LV* left ventricle, *RV* right ventricle)

▌ References

Aimé E, Frigiola A, Rovida M, Corno AF, De Ambroggi L (1993) Endomyocardial permanent pace-maker implantation in infants and children with postoperative a–v block. PACE 16:1143

Anderson RH, Lenox C, Zuberbuhler J (1983) Mechanisms of closure of perimembranous ventricular septal defect. Am J Cardiol 52:341–345

Campbell M (1971) Natural history of ventricular septal defect. Br Heart J 33:246

Cicini MP, Giannico S, Iorio FS, Giamberti A, Corno AF, Marino B, Marcelletti C (1990) Stenosi sottoaortica post-chirurgica dopo chiusura di difetto interventricolare. G Ital Cardiol 20(Suppl II):43

Cicini MP, Giannico S, Marino B, Iorio FS, Corno AF, Marcelletti C (1992) "Acquired" subvalvular aortic stenosis after repair of a ventricular septal defect. Chest 101:115–118

Corno AF, Marino B, Giamberti A, Latini L, Parisi F, Marcelletti C (1988) Difetti interventricolari sotto-arteriosi. Cardiol 33(Suppl II):138

Corno AF, Carta MG, Giannico S (1989) Pulmonary artery banding through median sternotomy. Cl Res 37:91A

Corno AF, Zoia E, Santoro F, Camesasca C, Biagioli B, Grossi A (1992) Epicardial damage induced by topical cooling during pediatric cardiac surgery. Br Heart J 67:174–176

Corno AF (1995) Congenital septal defects: role of the pulmonary artery banding on 1995. In: D'Alessandro LC (ed) Heart Surgery 1995. CESI, Rome, pp 167–175

Corno AF, von Segesser LK (1999) Is hypothermia necessary in pediatric cardiac surgery? Eur J Cardiothorac Surg 15:110–111

Corno AF (2000) Surgery for congenital heart disease. Curr Opinion Cardiol 15:238–243

De Leval MR, Pozzi M, Starnes V, Sullivan ID, Stark J, Somerville J, Anderson RH, Deanfield JE (1988) Surgical management of doubly committed subarterial ventricular septal defect. Circulation 78(Suppl III):40

Eroglu AG, Oztunc F, Saltik L, Bakari S, Dedeoglu S, Ahunbay G (2003) Evolution of ventricular septal defect with special reference to spontaneous closure rate, subaortic ridge and aortic valve prolapse. Pediatr Cardiol 24:31–35

Ferencz C, Rubin JD, McCarter RJ (1985) Congenital heart disease: prevalence at livebirth. The Baltimore-Washington infant study. Am J Epidemiol 121:31–36

Friedman WF, Mehrizi A, Pusch AL (1965) Multiple muscular ventricular septal defects. Circulation 32:35

Fyler DC, Buckley LP, Hellenbrand WE, Cohn HE (1980) Report of the New England Regional Infant Care Program. Pediatrics 65(Suppl):375–461

Gabriel HM, Heger M, Innerhofer P, Zehetgruber M, Mundigler G, Wimmer M, Maurer G, Baumgartner H (2002) Long-term outcome of patients with ventricular septal defect considered not to require surgical closure during childhood. J Am Coll Cardiol 20:1066–1071

Grabitz RG, Joffres MR, Collins-Nakai RL (1988) Congenital heart disease: incidence in the first year of life. The Alberta heritage pediatric cardiology program. Am J Epidemiol 128:381–388

Heath D, Edwards JE (1958) The pathology of hypertensive pulmonary vascular disease: a description of six grades of structural changes in the pulmonary arteries with special reference to congenital cardiac septal defects. Circulation 18:533

Hoffman JIE, Rudolph AM (1965) The natural history of ventricular septal defects in infancy. Am J Cardiol 16:634–653

Hoffman JIE, Kaplan S (2002) The incidence of congenital heart disease. J Am Coll Cardiol 39:1890–1900

Horisberger J, Jegger D, Boone Y, Seigneul I, Pierrel N, Hurni M, Corno AF, von Segesser LK (1999) Impact of a remote pump head on neonatal priming volumes. Perfusion 14:351–356

Kirklin JW, McGoon DC, DuShane JW (1960) Surgical treatment of ventricular septal defects. J Thorac Cardiovasc Surg 40:763

Kirklin JK, Castaneda AR, Keane JF, Fellows KE, Norwood WI (1980) Surgical management of multiple ventricular septal defects. J Thorac Cardiovasc Surg 80:458

Lillehei CW, Cohen M, Warden HE, Ziegler NR, Varco RL (1955) The result of direct vision closure of ventricular septal defects in eight patients by means of controlled cross circulation. Surg Gynecol Obstet 101:446

Marino B, Papa M, Guccione P, Corno AF, Marasini M, Calabrò R (1990) Ventricular septal defect in Down syndrome: anatomic types and associated malformations. Am J Dis Child 144:544–545

Marino B, Corno AF, Guccione P, Marcelletti C (1991) Ventricular septal defect and Down's syndrome. Lancet 337:245–246

Merrick AF, Lal M, Anderson RH, Shore DF (1999) Management of ventricular septal defect: a survey of practice in the United Kingdom. Ann Thorac Surg 68:983–988

Milella L, Da Cruz E, Gajraj RJ, Corno AF (1997) Computerized anaesthesia and normothermic perfusion in paediatric cardiac surgery. 2nd World Congress of Paediatric Cardiology and Cardiac Surgery, Abstracts, pp 376

Muller WH, Dammann JF (1952) The treatment of certain congenital malformations of the heart by the creation of pulmonic stenosis to reduce pulmonary hypertension and excessive pulmonary blood flow: a preliminary report. Surg Gynecol Obstet 95:213

Papa M, Santoro F, Corno AF (1993) Spontaneous closure of inlet ventricular septal defect in an infant with Down's syndrome and aortic coarctation. Chest 104:620–622

Pongiglione G, Freedom RM, Cook D, Rowe R (1982) Mechanism of acquired right ventricular outflow tract obstruction in patients with ventricular septal defect: an angiographic study. Am J Cardiol 50:776–780

Singh AK, de Leval MR, Stark J (1977) Left ventriculotomy for closure of muscular ventricular septal defects. Ann Surg 186:577

Somerville J, Brandao A, Ross DN (1970) Aortic regurgitation with ventricular septal defect. Circulation 41:317–330

Trusler GA, Mustard WT (1972) A method of banding the pulmonary artery for large isolated ventricular septal defect with and without transposition of the great arteries. Ann Thorac Surg 13:351

Trusler GA, Moes CAF, Kidd BSL (1973) Repair of ventricular septal defect with aortic insufficiency. J Thorac Cardiovasc Surg 66:394

Tsang VT, Hsia TY, Yates RW, Anderson RH (2002) Surgical repair of supposedly multiple defects within the apical part of the muscular ventricular septum. Ann Thorac Surg 73:58–62

Turner SW, Hornung T, Hunter S (2002) Closure of ventricular septal defects: a study of factors influencing spontaneous and surgical closure. Cardiol Young 12:357–363

Wagenvoort CA, Neufeld HN, DuShane JW, Edwards JE (1961) The pulmonary arterial tree in ventricular septal defect: a quantitative study of anatomic features in fetuses, infants and children. Circulation 23:740

▮ Incidence

Tetralogy of Fallot is the 5th most common congenital heart defect. This occurs in about 0.19–0.26/1000 live births. It constitutes 6.8% of all congenital heart diseases. It is the most common cyanotic congenital heart disease beyond 1 week of age.

▮ Morphology (Figs. 1.7.1 and 1.7.2)

In anatomic terms the malformation is composed of four constant features: subpulmonary infundibular stenosis, ventricular septal defect, rightward deviation of the aortic valve with biventricular origin of its leaflets, hypertrophy of the wall of the right ventricle (Fig. 1.7.3).

Although all hearts have comparable features, the malformation represents a morphological spectrum, with one morphological hallmark which unifies the overall entity: the antero-cephalad deviation of the infundibular septum, the muscular structure which separates the subaortic and pulmonary outlets, relative to the rest of the muscular septum.

Although unified in the sense of the septal malalignment, the patients with tetralogy of Fallot have significant variations in the precise anatomy of the ventricular septal defect, the nature of pulmonary infundibular and valvular stenosis, and the degree of aortic override which account for the differences in hemodynamic consequences.

The ventricular septal defect is located in the membranous septum; it is subaortic and

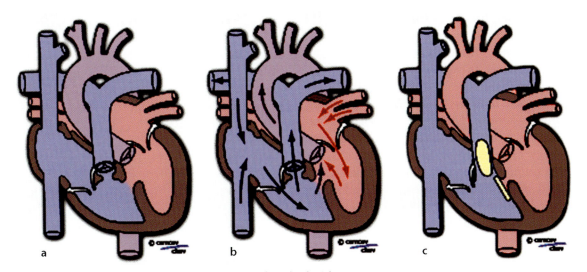

Fig. 1.7.1. Tetralogy of Fallot: mild form. **a** morphology, **b** pathophysiology, **c** surgery

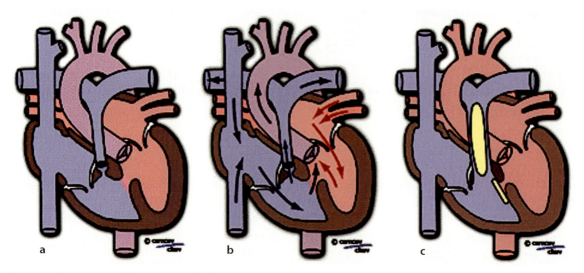

Fig. 1.7.2. Tetralogy of Fallot: severe infundibular obstruction, small pulmonary valve annulus and main pulmonary artery. **a** morphology, **b** pathophysiology, **c** surgery

sometimes extends to the subpulmonic valve area. The ventricular septal defect is large, at least as the aortic valve, causing equalization of left and right ventricular pressures. These defects do not usually become smaller and are not known to close spontaneously. The right ventricular outflow tract is hypoplastic and almost always obstructive. Occasionally at birth the right ventricular outflow tract shows no significant obstruction and results in the so-called "pink" tetralogy of Fallot. The pulmonary valve annulus is typically small in tetralogy of Fallot and the leaflets are deformed. The main pulmonary artery as well as the branch pulmonary arteries are small in contrast to pulmonary valvular stenosis. There might be branch pulmonary artery stenosis as well as peripheral pulmonary artery stenosis in addition to the right ventricular outflow tract and pulmonary valvular stenosis. Bronchial arterial collaterals which connect to the peripheral pulmonary arteries are sometimes present. The main pulmonary artery is occasionally atretic and the pulmonary arteries are fed either by patent ductus arteriosus or collateral vessels. The aortic valve is typically large.

▌ Associated anomalies

Atrial septal defect or patent foramen ovale (frequent, 40% of the patients), anomalous pulmonary venous connection (rare), persistent left superior vena cava, supravalvular mitral stenosis (rare), cor triatriatum (rare), atrioventricular septal defect, multiple ventricular septal defects, restrictive ventricular septal defect (rare), hypoplastic or absent infundibular septum, fibromuscular subaortic stenosis (rare), valvular aortic stenosis (rare), valvular aortic regurgitation, anomalous coronary arteries (frequent, 10% of the patients), right aortic arch (frequent, 25% of the patients), aorto-pulmonary window, patent ductus arteriosus, aortic coarctation (rare), vascular ring, non-confluent pulmonary arteries, anomalous origin of the left subclavian artery, major aorto-pulmonary collateral arteries.

▌ Pathophysiology

Progressive anatomic and dynamic right ventricular outflow tract obstruction, with bidirectional or right-to-left shunt at the ventricular level, depending on the degree of the infundibular and/or pulmonary valve

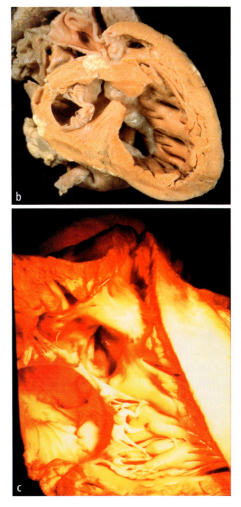

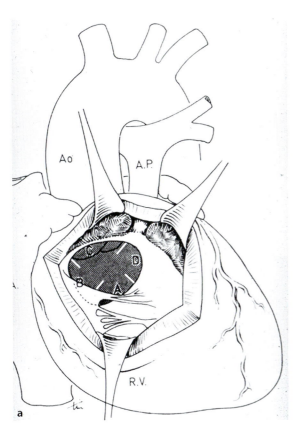

Fig. 1.7.3. Tetralogy of Fallot: morphology. **a** schema showing the four constant features: subpulmonary infundibular stenosis, ventricular septal defect, rightward deviation of the aortic valve with biventricular origin of its leaflets, hypertrophy of the wall of the right ventricle (*Ao* aorta, *AP* pulmonary artery, *RV* right ventricle), **b** photograph showing the four constant features: subpulmonary infundibular stenosis, ventricular septal defect, rightward deviation of the aortic valve with biventricular origin of its leaflets, hypertrophy of the wall of the right ventricle, **c** transilluminated photograph showing the four constant features: subpulmonary infundibular stenosis, ventricular septal defect, rightward deviation of the aortic valve with biventricular origin of its leaflets, hypertrophy of the wall of the right ventricle (photograph courtesy of Dr. S.Y. Ho)

stenosis; systemic right ventricular pressure, due to the presence of the unrestrictive ventricular septal defect, reduced pulmonary artery pressure and pulmonary blood flow.

▪ Diagnosis

The right ventricular outflow tract obstruction may be minimal in the beginning leading to significant left-to-right shunting at the ventricular septal defect with symptoms and signs of congestive heart failure. As the right ventricular outflow tract becomes more and more obstructive the pulmonary vascular resistance will exceed the systemic vascular resistance and right-to-left shunting will occur causing cyanosis.

Cyanosis is influenced by hemoglobin level; thus if low cyanosis may not be evident. Cyanosis induces an increase in the hemoglobin concentration and increase in erythropoietin production. When there are large or multiple collaterals from the systemic arterial circulation to the pulmonary arterial circulation, there is minimal cyanosis as pulmonary blood flow is increased.

Only 25% of tetralogy of Fallot patients are cyanotic at birth, while 75% of patients become cyanotic at 1 year of age. Hypoxic spells are more rare in the first six months of life, and they are most common in infants and toddlers; they again become rare in children more than 4 years of age.

Squatting helps to relieve cyanotic spells possibly due to increase in systemic vascular resistance because of kinking of femoral arteries as well as in a decrease in the venous return.

The long systolic murmur of tetralogy of Fallot is secondary to the turbulent flow across the right ventricular outflow tract obstruction and pulmonary stenosis and not due to the ventricular septal defect. Due to deformity of the pulmonary valve, there may be a single second heart sound. When continuous murmurs are auscultated this might indicate the presence of a patent ductus arteriosus or collateral vessels.

■ **Clinical pattern:** clinical presentation depends on the degree of pulmonary stenosis; usually progressive cyanosis in infancy, with hypoxic (hypercyanotic) spells.

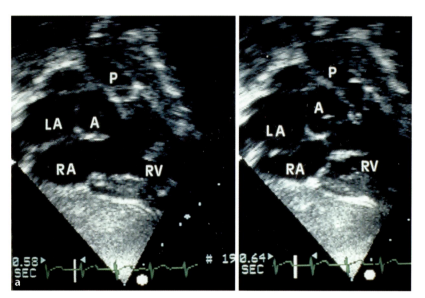

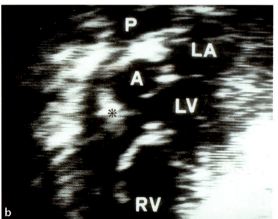

Fig. 1.7.4. Tetralogy of Fallot: echocardiography. **a** right oblique view showing the large perimembranous ventricular septal defect with associated anterior and rightward deviation of the infundibular septum, resulting in the overriding of the aortic valve on the interventricular septum and right ventricular outflow tract obstruction, **b** left oblique view showing the large perimembranous ventricular septal defect with associated anterior and rightward deviation of the infundibular septum, resulting in the overriding of the aortic valve on the interventricular septum and right ventricular outflow tract obstruction (*A* aorta, *LA* left atrium, *P* pulmonary artery, *RA* right atrium, *RV* right ventricle, asterisk = deviated infundibular septum) (reproduced with permission from Marino B, Thiene G (1990) Atlante di anatomia ecocardiografica delle cardiopatie congenite, USES, Firenze)

■ **Electrocardiogram:** right axis deviation, right ventricular hypertrophy.

■ **Chest X-ray:** lung hypoperfusion, absent or small pulmonary artery segment (= boot shape), elevated cardiac apex, mild (if any) cardiac enlargement.

■ **Echocardiogram:** large perimembranous ventricular septal defect with associated anterior and rightward deviation of the infundibular septum, resulting in the overriding of the aortic valve on the interventricular septum; this anterior deviation is responsible in large part for the right ventricular outflow tract obstruction (Fig. 1.7.4); the coronary arteries pattern can be identified by echocardiography; in patients with classic anatomy, without associated cardiac malformations, the palliative and the corrective surgery may be guided by echocardiography alone.

■ **Cardiac catheterization:** indication for cardiac catheterization is guided by the surgical management strategy; the following information is required (Fig. 1.7.5):
- number, size and location of all ventricular septal defects,
- site(s) and severity of right ventricular outflow tract obstruction,
- size and distribution of pulmonary arteries,
- pattern of coronary artery origins and branching,
- origin and distribution of all additional sources of pulmonary blood flow, particularly anatomy and distribution of major aorto-pulmonary collateral arteries when present.

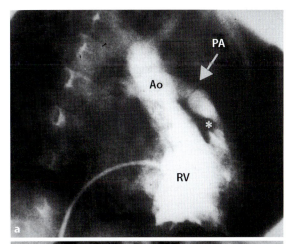
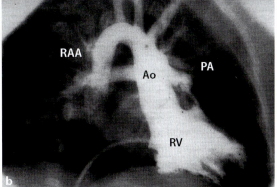
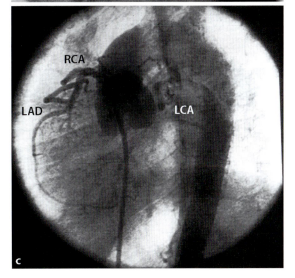

Fig. 1.7.5. Tetralogy of Fallot: angiography. **a** Right ventricular injection showing opacification of the ascending aorta through the ventricular septal defect and infundibular and valvular pulmonary stenosis (*Ao* aorta, *PA* pulmonary artery, *RV* right ventricle, asterisk = deviated infundibular septum), **b** right ventricular injection showing opacification of the ascending aorta through the ventricular septal defect, severe infundibular and valvular pulmonary stenosis, and right aortic arch (*RAA* right aortic arch), **c** contrast injection showing opacification of the ascending aorta with the left anterior descending (LAD) coronary artery originating from the right coronary artery (RCA) (*LCA* left coronary artery)

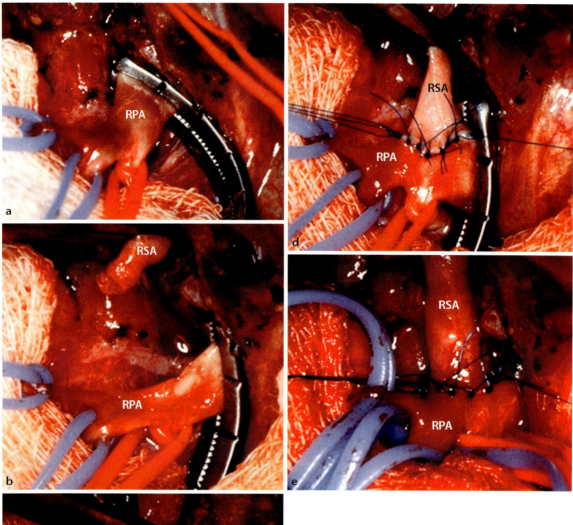

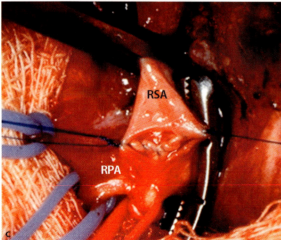

Fig. 1.7.6. Tetralogy of Fallot: classic right Blalock-Taussig shunt. **a** the right pulmonary artery (RPA) is dissected free and then controlled proximally with a vascular clamp and distally with elastic vessel-loops, **b** the prepared and transected right subclavian artery (RSA) is approximated to the right pulmonary artery (RPA), opened with a transversal incision, **c** the posterior wall of the right subclavian artery (RSA), controlled with a vascular clamp, is end-to-side anastomosed to the right pulmonary artery (RPA) with a running suture, **d** the anterior wall of the right subclavian artery (RSA) is anastomosed to the right pulmonary artery (RPA) with interrupted sutures, **e** the elastic vessel-loops are released and the vascular clamps are removed, providing lung perfusion

■ Indications for surgical treatment

■ **Cyanotic spells:** these typically occur when babies or toddlers are upset leading to an increase in the catecholamines and consequently an increase in the right ventricular outflow tract obstruction and more right-to-left shunting at the ventricular septal defect level. The first line of treatment should be to ask a parent to hold and comfort the child, usually this will break the spell. When holding the child it is best to place him in the knee-chest position to increase the systemic vascular resistance.

When this fails then one might utilize one of the following measures:

■ morphine subcutaneously or intravenously to cause a negative inotropic response and to reduce the right-to-left shunt by reducing the right ventricular outflow tract obstruction; in addition, it has a sedative analgesic effect that might cause the child to relax, resulting in a lower catecholamine level and less right ventricular outflow tract obstruction;

■ beta blockers such as intravenous or intramuscular Inderal to cause a negative inotropic effect and less right ventricular outflow tract obstruction, thus breaking the cyanotic spell;

■ peripheral vasoconstrictors such as a drip of epinephrine or phenylephrine hydrochloride to cause systemic vasoconstriction and elevation of the systemic vascular resistance with less right-to-left shunting.

■ Patients *asymptomatic or with very mild cyanosis*: surgical repair between 1 and 2 years of age.

■ Patients with *significant hypoxemia or hypercyanotic spells*: surgical repair at the time of presentation, regardless of age.

■ Infants with *associated anomalies* (major anomalous coronary artery crossing the

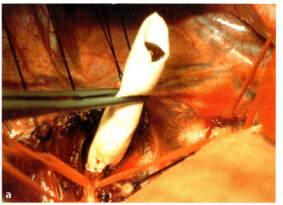

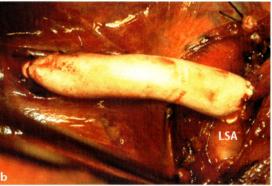

Fig. 1.7.7. Tetralogy of Fallot: modified left Blalock-Taussig shunt. **a** the distal end of a PTFE tubular prosthesis is end-to-side anastomosed to the left pulmonary artery, controlled with elastic vessel loops, **b** the proximal end of the PTFE tubular prosthesis is end-to-side anastomosed to the left subclavian artery

infundibulum, multiple ventricular septal defects, atrio-ventricular septal defect, hypoplastic left ventricle): palliative treatment by means of a systemic-to-pulmonary artery shunt: classical (Fig. 1.7.6) or modified (Fig. 1.7.7) Blalock-Taussig anastomosis.

■ Infants with *significant hypoplasia of the distal branch pulmonary arteries*, but with right ventricle-pulmonary artery continuity: right ventricular outflow tract reconstruction, with or without perforated ventricular septal defect patch (for subsequent cardiac catheterization closure).

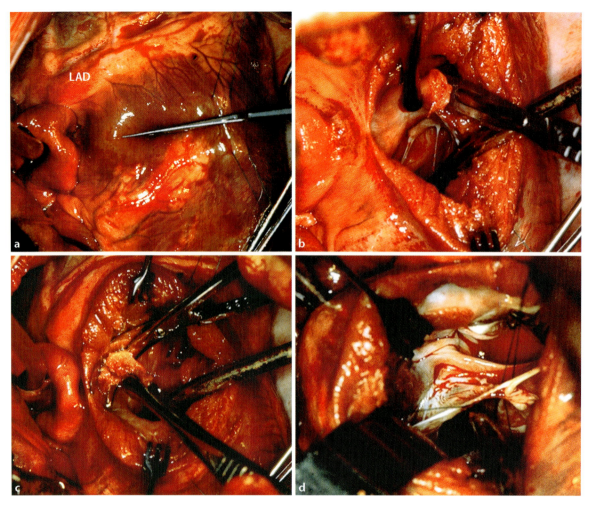

Fig. 1.7.8. Tetralogy of Fallot: transventricular repair. **a** longitudinal right ventriculotomy, parallel to the left anterior descending (LAD) coronary artery, **b** after retraction of the edges of the longitudinal right ventriculotomy, knife resection of the infundibulum, **c** completion with scissors of the infundibular resection to relieve the right ventricular outflow tract obstruction at the level of the infundibulum, **d** exposure of the ventricular septal defect, with the interrupted pledgeted sutures to be utilized for patch closure of the defect already through the septal leaflet of the tricuspid valve, **e** prosthetic patch for closure of the ventricular septal defect anastomosed to the septal leaflet of the tricuspid valve with the interrupted pledgeted sutures, **f** prosthetic patch for closure of the ventricular septal defect anastomosed to the rest of the rim of the defect with running sutures, **g** prosthetic patch closure of the ventricular septal defect almost completed, leaving the aortic valve on the left ventricular side, **h** enlargement of the right ventricular outflow tract by closure of the right ventriculotomy with transannular pericardial patch (TPP)

▮ Surgical treatment (on cardiopulmonary bypass)

▮ *Patch closure of the ventricular septal defect* from the transatrial-transpulmonary or from transventricular approach with longitudinal ventriculotomy (Fig. 1.7.8).
▮ *Right ventricular outflow tract reconstruction:*

– from the right atrium and/or from the pulmonary artery (transatrial-transpulmonary approach) or from the right ventricle (transventricular approach): incision with resection of the heavy trabeculations that bind the infundibular septum to the anterior right ventricular wall;

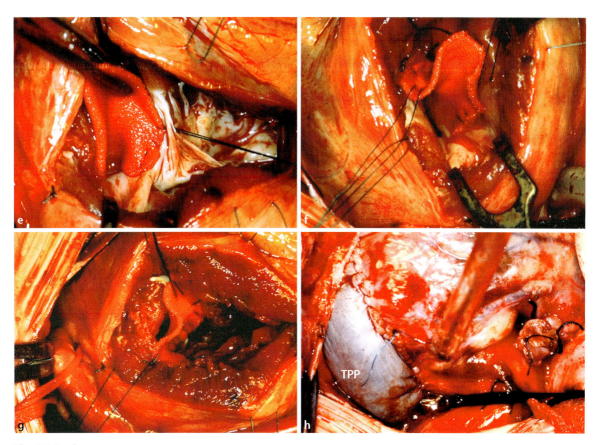

Fig. 1.7.8 e–h

– infundibular (pericardial or synthetic) patch enlargement (transventricular approach);
– transannular (pericardial or synthetic, with or without monocusp) patch enlargement (transatrial-transpulmonary and transventricular approach) in case of inadequate size of the pulmonary valve annulus, measured with Hegar dilators, after pulmonary valvotomy performed from the pulmonary artery (transatrial-transpulmonary approach) or from the right ventricle (transventricular approach);
– pulmonary arteries enlargement in case of inadequate size (measured with Hegar dilators), with prolongation of the transannular patch in case of inadequate left pulmonary artery, with separate patch in case of inadequate right pulmonary artery;

– valved conduit, generally biologic, interposed between the right ventriculotomy and the pulmonary artery bifurcation, to bypass an anomalous coronary artery (Fig. 1.7.9).

▮ Potential complications

▮ *Palliative treatment (systemic-to-pulmonary artery shunt):* Inadequate pulmonary blood flow (insufficient, excessive or disomogeneous), pulmonary artery distortion, inadequate growth of the pulmonary arteries, acquired pulmonary atresia.

▮ *Repair:* Residual or recurrent ventricular septal defect (patch dehiscence or separate defect), residual or recurrent right ventricular outflow tract obstruction, complete atrioventricular block, arrhythmias,

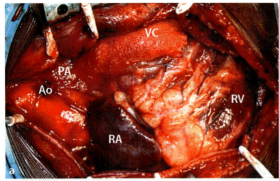

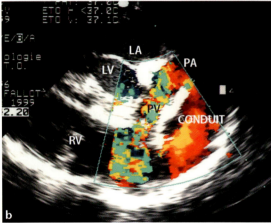

Fig. 1.7.9. Tetralogy of Fallot: right ventricle to pulmonary artery valved conduit. **a** intra-operative photograph showing the valved conduit implanted between the right ventricle and pulmonary artery (*Ao* aorta, *PA* pulmonary artery, *RA* right atrium, *RV* right ventricle, *VC* valved conduit), **b** post-operative transesophageal echocardiography with color Doppler showing the iatrogenic double outlet from the right ventricle, with flow through the native stenotic outlet and from the valved conduit implanted between the right ventricle and pulmonary artery (*CONDUIT* valved conduit, *LA* left atrium, *LV* left ventricle, *RA* pulmonary artery, *PV* pulmonary valve, *RV* right ventricle) (Photograph courtesy of Dr. Pierre-Guy Chassot)

aneurysm of right ventricular outflow patch, pulmonary valve insufficiency.

∎ *Late complications:*
- pulmonary valve regurgitation:
  long standing pulmonary valve regurgitation, particularly after repair with transannular patch enlargement, can determine right ventricular dilatation and failure, with or without subsequent tricuspid valve regurgitation, requiring for reoperation the insertion of a valve

or a biological valve conduit in the pulmonary valve position;
- arrhythmias:
  supraventricular and ventricular arrhythmias can occur years after repair, requiring electrophysiology or pacemaker insertion.

∎ **References**

Alexiou C, Chen Q, Galogavrou M, Gnanapragasam J, Salmon AP, Keeton BR, Haw MP, Monro JL (2002) Repair of tetralogy of Fallot in infancy with a transventricular or a transatrial approach. Eur J Cardiothorac Surg 22:174–183

Anderson RH, Allwork SP, Ho SY, Lenox CC, Zuberbuhler JR (1981) Surgical anatomy of tetralogy of Fallot. J Thorac Cardiovasc Surg 81:887–896

Barnard CN, Schrire V (1961) The surgical treatment of the tetralogy of Fallot. Thorax 16:346

Blalock A, Taussig HB (1945) The surgical treatment of malformations of the heart in which there is pulmonary stenosis or pulmonary atresia. JAMA 128:189–192

Brock RC, Campbell M (1950) Infundibular resection or dilatation for infundibular stenosis. Br Heart J 12:403

Castaneda AR, Freed MD, Williams RG, Norwood WI (1977) Repair of tetralogy of Fallot in infancy. Early and late results. J Thorac Cardiovasc Surg 74:372–381

Cobanoglu A, Schultz JM (2002) Total correction of tetralogy of Fallot in the first year of life: late results. Ann Thorac Surg 74:133–138

Corno AF, Giamberti A, Giannico S, Marino B, Picardo S, Ballerini L, Marcelletti C (1988) Long-term results after extracardiac valved conduits implanted for complex congenital heart disease. J Card Surg 3:495–500

Corno AF, Giamberti A, Giannico S, Marino B, Rossi E, Marcelletti C, Kirklin JK (1990) Airway obstruction associated with congenital heart disease in infancy. J Thorac Cardiovasc Surg 99:1091–1098

Corno AF, Zoia E, Santoro F, Camesasca C, Biagioli B, Grossi A (1992) Epicardial damage induced by topical cooling during pediatric cardiac surgery. Br Heart J 67:174–176

Corno AF (1993) Rare cardiac malformations. In: D'Alessandro LC (ed) Heart Surgery 1993. CESI, Rome, pp 189–199

Corno AF, Da Cruz E, Milella L, Wilson N (1997) Controlled reoxygenation for cyanotic patients. 2nd World Congress of Paediatric Cardiology and Cardiac Surgery, Abstracts, p 186

Corno AF, Da Cruz E, Lal AB, Milella L, Wilson N (1998) Controlled reoxygenation for cyanotic patients. In: Imai Y, Momma K (eds) Proceedings of 2nd World Congress of PCCS. Futura Publishing Co., Armonk, NY, pp 1127–1129

Corno AF, Hurni M, Payot M, von Segesser LK (1999) Modified Blalock-Taussig shunt with compensatory properties. Ann Thorac Surg 67:269–270

Corno AF, von Segesser LK (1999) Is hypothermia necessary in pediatric cardiac surgery? Eur J Cardiothorac Surg 15:110–111

Corno AF (2000) Surgery for congenital heart disease. Curr Opinion Cardiol 15:238–243

Corno AF, Hurni M, Griffin H, Galal OM, Payot M, Sekarski N, Tozzi P, von Segesser LK (2002) Bovine jugular vein as right ventricle-to-pulmonary artery valved conduit. J Heart Valve Dis 11:242–247

Dabizzi RP, Caprioli G, Aiazzi L (1980) Distribution and anomalies of the coronary arteries in tetralogy of Fallot. Circulation 61:95–102

Da Cruz E, Milella L, Corno AF (1998) Left isomerism with tetralogy of Fallot and anomalous systemic and pulmonary venous connections. Cardiol Young 8:131–133

Davlouros PA, Kilner PJ, Hornung TS, Li W, Francis JM, Moon JCC, Smith GC, Tat T, Pennell DJ, Gatzoulis MA (2002) Right ventricular function in adults with repaired tetralogy of Fallot assessed with cardiovascular magnetic resonance imaging: detrimental role of right ventricular outflow aneurysm or akinesia and adverse right-to-left ventricular interaction. J Am Coll Cardiol 40:2044–2052

De Leval MR, McKay R, Jones M, Stark J, Macartney FJ (1981) Modified Blalock-Taussig shunt. Use of subclavian artery orifice as flow regulator in prosthetic systemic-pulmonary shunts. J Thorac Cardiovasc Surg 81:112

De Ruijter FT, Weenink I, Hitchcock FJ, Meijboom EJ, Bennink GB (2002) Right ventricular dysfunction and pulmonary valve replacement after correction of tetralogy of Fallot. Ann Thorac Surg 73:1794–1800

Ebert PA (1982) Second operation for pulmonary stenosis or insufficiency after repair of tetralogy of Fallot. Am J Cardiol 50:637

Edmunds LH, Saxena NC, Friedman S, Rashkind WJ, Dodd PF (1976) Transatrial repair of tetralogy of Fallot. Surgery 80:681

Fallot A (1888) Contribution à l'anatomie pathologique de la maladie bleue (cyanose cardiaque). Marseille Med 25:77–83

Ferencz C, Rubin JD, McCarter RJ (1985) Congenital heart disease: prevalence at livebirth. The Baltimore-Washington infant study. Am J Epidemiol 121:31–36

Fyler DC, Buckley LP, Hellenbrand WE, Cohn HE (1980) Report of the New England Regional Infant Care Program. Pediatrics 65(Suppl):375–461

Ghai A, Silversides C, Harris L, Webb GD, Siu SC, Therrien J (2002) Left ventricular dysfunction is a risk factor for sudden cardiac death in adults late after repair of tetralogy of Fallot. J Am Coll Cardiol 40:1675–1680

Giannopoulos NM, Chatzis AK, Karros P, Zavaropoulos P, Papagiannis J, Rammos S, Kirvassilis GV, Sarris GE (2002) Early results after transatrial/transpulmonary repair of tetralogy of Fallot. Eur J Cardiothorac Surg 22:582–586

Giomarelli P, Biagioli B, Lisi G, Santoro F, Corno AF (1989) On-line metabolic and ventilatory monitoring in pediatric cardiac operation. J Thorac Cardiovasc Surg 97:939–940

Giomarelli P, Biagioli B, Rosi R, Simeone F, Santoro F, Lisi G, Corno AF (1989) Postoperative on-line ventilatory monitoring in pediatric patients after palliative or corrective procedure for tetralogy of Fallot. Cuore 6:463–468

Gootman NL, Scarpelli EM, Rudolph AM (1963) Metabolic acidosis in children with severe cyanotic congenital heart disease. Pediatrics 31:251–254

Hoffman JIE, Kaplan S (2002) The incidence of congenital heart disease. J Am Coll Cardiol 39:1890–1900

Hurni M, Corno AF, Tucker OP, Payot M, Sekarski N, Cotting J, Bernath MA, von Segesser LK (2000) Venpro: a new pulmonary valved conduit. Thorac Cardiovasc Surg 48(Suppl I):120

Kirklin JW, Ellis FH, McGoon DC, DuShane JW, Swan HFC (1959) Surgical treatment for tetralogy of Fallot by open intracardiac repair. J Thorac Surg 37:22

Lev M, Rimoldi HJA, Rowlatt DF (1964) Quantitative anatomy of cyanotic tetralogy of Fallot. Circulation 30:531

Lillehei CW, Cohen M, Warden HE, Read RC, Aust JB, De Wall RA, Varco RL (1955) Direct vision intracardiac surgical correction of the tetralogy of Fallot, pentalogy of Fallot, and pulmonary atresia defects: report of first ten cases. Ann Surg 142:418

Marcelletti C, Corno F, Losekoot TG, Olthof H, Schuller J, Bulterijs AHK, Becker AE (1980) Condotti extracardiaci: indicazioni, tecniche e risultati immediati. G Ital Cardiol 10:1041–1054

Marcelletti C, Corno AF (1981) Extracardiac conduits: indications, techniques and early results. 33th Herhalings Cursus Kindergeneeskunde, Amsterdam (Abstracts)

Marino B, Corno AF, Pasquini L, Guccione P, Carta MG, Ballerini L, De Simone G, Marcelletti C (1987) Indication for systemic-pulmonary artery shunts guided by two-dimensional and Doppler echocardiography: criteria for patient selection. Ann Thorac Surg 44:495–498

Marino B, Giannico S, Pasquini L, Corno AF, Picardo S (1988) Balloon-occlusion of the carotid artery for the angiographic visualization of Blalock-Taussig shunts and pulmonary arteries. Chest 94:267–269

Marino B, Corno AF, Carotti A, Pasquini L, Giannico S, Guccione P, Bevilacqua M, De Simone G, Marcelletti C (1990) Pediatric cardiac surgery guided by echocardiography. Scand J Thorac Cardiovasc Surg 24:197–201

Therrien J, Marx GR, Gatzoulis MA (2002) Late problems in tetralogy of Fallot: recognition, management and prevention. Cardiol Clin 20:395–404

Uebing A, Fischer G, Bethge M, Scheewe J, Schmiel F, Stich J, Brossman J, Kramer HH (2002) Influence of the pulmonary annulus diameter on pulmonary regurgitation and right ventricular pressure load after repair of tetralogy of Fallot. Heart 88:510–514

Van Doorn C (2002) The unnatural history of tetralogy of Fallot: surgical repair is not as definitive as previously thought. Heart 88:447–448

Van Praagh R, Van Praagh S, Nebesar RA, Muster AJ, Sinha SN, Paul MH (1970) Tetralogy of Fallot: underdevelopment of the pulmonary infundibulum and its sequelae. Am J Cardiol 26:25–33

Van Praagh R (1990) Etienne-Louis Arthur Fallot and his tetralogy: a new translation of Fallot's summary and a modern reassessment of this anomaly. Eur J Cardiothorac Surg 4:231–232

Tetralogy of Fallot with absent pulmonary valve

Incidence

Tetralogy of Fallot with absent pulmonary valve is a very rare malformation.

Morphology

This is an uncommon variation of tetralogy of Fallot.

There is a ring-like and usually stenotic malformation (rather than absence) of the pulmonary valve, with failure of the development of valve cusps; usually the pulmonary valve leaflets are mere myxomatous nubbins of valvar tissue.

The central pulmonary arteries are usually extremely dilated or aneurysmal. The pulmonary artery dilatation may extend beyond what is expected from severe pulmonary regurgitation to several generations of pulmonary arteries causing tracheobronchial compression; this often results in either hyperexpansion from air trapping or collapse of lobes, or even an entire lung.

The ductus arteriosus is generally absent.

The intracardiac anatomy generally presents with the same characteristics of tetralogy of Fallot (see chapter "Tetralogy of Fallot"), except that the right ventricular outflow tract is not excessively restrictive.

Associated anomalies

Atrial septal defect, common atrio-ventricular valve (rare), tricuspid atresia (rare), intact ventricular septum (rare), transposition of the great arteries (rare), agenesis of the ductus arteriosus, branch pulmonary arteries anomalies (non-confluent pulmonary arteries), right aortic arch (frequent), anomalous coronary arteries, dextrocardia and situs inversus (very rare).

Pathophysiology

Combination of the pathophysiologic pattern of tetralogy of Fallot (progressive dynamic right ventricular outflow tract obstruction, with a right-to-left or bidirectional shunt at the ventricular level, depending on the degree of the infundibular and/or pulmonary valve stenosis) with airway obstruction due to bronchial compression by the dilated pulmonary artery.

Diagnosis

The clinical picture is dominated by pulmonary regurgitation rather than pulmonary stenosis.

A systolic and diastolic murmur is present; this represents pulmonary stenosis and pulmonary regurgitation.

Clinical pattern: the clinical manifestations may be pulmonary, cardiac, or both (frequently); the patients are categorized into two well-defined groups:
1) infants (frequently neonates) with severe respiratory symptoms of tachypnea, bronchospasm, air trapping, cyanosis or actual respiratory failure;
2) older children with less severe symptoms.

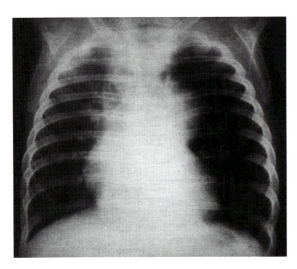

Fig. 1.8.1. Tetralogy of Fallot with absent pulmonary valve: chest X-ray. Marked supracardiac mediastinal widening because of aneurysmal dilatation of the pulmonary artery, with relatively oligemic lung fields; aerated portions of the left lung overinflated

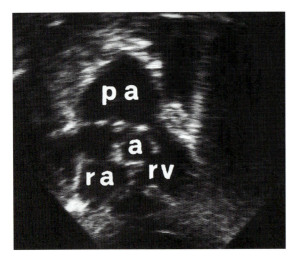

Fig. 1.8.2. Tetralogy of Fallot with absent pulmonary valve: echocardiography. Right oblique view with subaortic ventricular septal defect, obstruction of the right ventricular outflow tract with small pulmonary valve annulus and the huge dilatation of the main pulmonary artery (*a* aorta, *pa* pulmonary artery, *ra* right atrium, *rv* right ventricle)

▮ **Electrocardiogram:** right axis deviation, right atrial enlargement, right ventricular hypertrophy.

▮ **Chest X-ray:** diagnostic in most cases (Fig. 1.8.1); marked supracardiac mediastinal widening (aneurysmal dilatation of pulmonary arteries), with relatively oligemic lung fields; segmental or lobar atelectasis is common; the aerated portions of lung may be overinflated (obstructive emphysema).

▮ **Echocardiogram:** intracardiac anatomy: same as for tetralogy of Fallot, but with very dilated main pulmonary artery segment and central pulmonary arteries (Fig. 1.8.2); Doppler examination shows a grossly incompetent pulmonary valve.

▮ **Cardiac catheterization:** useful to provide definition of the degree of aneurysmal dilatation of the main and branch pulmonary arteries (Fig. 1.8.3), important to delineate the peripheral pulmonary arteries and to rule out additional lesions: anomalous coronary arteries, multiple ventricular septal defects; this investigation can be associated with tracheobronchography (Fig. 1.8.4) of tracheobronchofibroscopy to identify obstructions of the airways.

▮ Indications for surgical treatment

The timing of surgery relates to the severity of symptoms; neonates and infants generally require urgent repair because of respiratory symptoms, older children are able to wait for elective repair.

Management is delayed as much as possible because of the need to place a valved conduit, usually a homograft or heterograft.

Surgery is done earlier in patients with dilated distal pulmonary arteries and respiratory distress to halt further progress of bronchoconstriction.

Pulmonary arteries need to be plicated during surgery.

Hypercyanotic spells are not a feature of this type of tetralogy of Fallot.

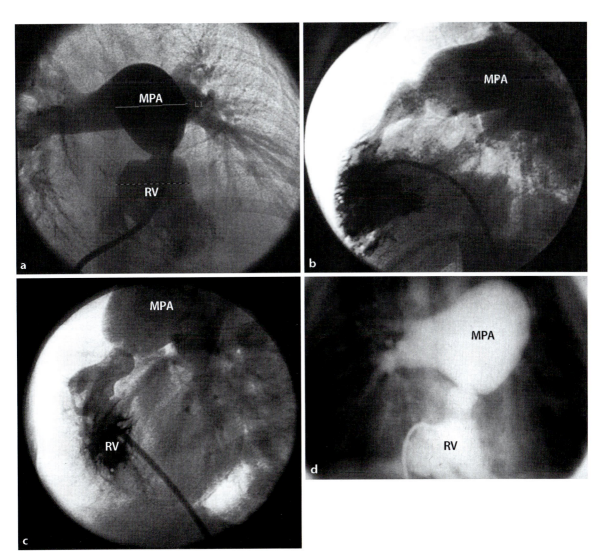

Fig. 1.8.3. Tetralogy of Fallot with absent pulmonary valve: angiography. **a** antero-posterior projection, showing the dilation of the main and branch pulmonary arteries (*MPA* main pulmonary artery, *RV* right ventricle), **b** lateral projection with right ventricular injection showing the right ventricular outflow tract obstruction and the dilation of the main and branch pulmonary arteries, **c** left oblique projection with right ventricular injection showing the aneurysmal dilation of the main pulmonary artery, **d** antero-posterior projection, showing the dilation of the main and branch pulmonary arteries (reproduced with permission from Corno AF, Picardo S, Ballerini L, Gugliantini P, Marcelletti C (1985) Bronchial compression by dilated pulmonary artery: surgical treatment. J Thorac Cardiovasc Surg 90:706–720)

▮ Surgical treatment (on cardiopulmonary bypass)

Excision of the main pulmonary artery, with transection of its proximal end just above the pulmonary valve annulus and of its distal end at the level of the bifurcation. Resection and plication of the aneurysmal pulmonary arteries, extended laterally to the hilum, with or without including the plication of the posterior wall of both pulmonary arteries. Transannular longitudinal right ventriculotomy. Patch closure of the ventricular septal defect from a longitudinal right ventriculotomy. Valved conduit (homograft or heterograft) interposition between the right ventricle and the reconstructed pulmonary arteries bifurcation.

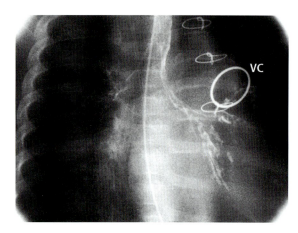

Fig. 1.8.4. Tetralogy of Fallot with absent pulmonary valve: tracheobronchography. Post-operative investigation (in the same patient of Fig. 1.8.3 d), after repair with implantation of a valved conduit (with a metal ring corresponding to the biological valve) between the right ventricle and pulmonary artery, showing the residual subtotal occlusion of the left main bronchus (reproduced with permission from Corno AF, Picardo S, Ballerini L, Gugliantini P, Marcelletti C (1985) Bronchial compression by dilated pulmonary artery: surgical treatment. J Thorac Cardiovasc Surg 90:706–720)

▮ Potential complications

Residual or recurrent ventricular septal defect (patch dehiscence or separate defect), residual or recurrent right ventricular outflow tract obstruction, complete atrioventricular block, arrhythmias, airway compression, respiratory insufficiency.

▮ References

Corno AF, Picardo S, Ballerini L, Gugliantini P, Marcelletti C (1985) Bronchial compression by dilated pulmonary artery: surgical treatment. J Thorac Cardiovasc Surg 90:706–720

Corno AF, Giamberti A, Giannico S, Marino B, Picardo S, Ballerini L, Marcelletti C (1988) Long-term results after extracardiac valved conduits implanted for complex congenital heart disease. J Card Surg 3:495–500

Corno AF, Giamberti A, Giannico S, Marino B, Rossi E, Marcelletti C, Kirklin JK (1990) Airway obstruction associated with congenital heart disease in infancy. J Thorac Cardiovasc Surg 99:1091–1098

Corno AF, von Segesser LK (1999) Is hypothermia necessary in pediatric cardiac surgery? Eur J Cardiothorac Surg 15:110–111

Corno AF, Hurni M, Griffin H, Galal OM, Payot M, Sekarski N, Tozzi P, von Segesser LK (2002) Bovine jugular vein as right ventricle-to-pulmonary artery valved conduit. J Heart Valve Dis 11:242–247

Hew CC, Daebritz SH, Zurakowski D, del Nido PI, Mayer JE, Jonas RA (2002) Valved homograft replacement of aneurysmal pulmonary arteries for severely symptomatic absent pulmonary valve syndrome. Ann Thorac Surg 73:1778–1785

Hiraishi S, Bargeron LM, Isabel-Jones JB, Emmanouilides GC, Friedman WF, Jarmakani JM (1983) Ventricular and pulmonary artery volumes in patients with absent pulmonary valve. Factors affecting the natural course. Circulation 67:183

Hraska V, Kantorova A, Kunovsky P, Haviar D (2002) Intermediate results with correction of tetralogy of Fallot with absent pulmonary valve using a new approach. Eur J Cardiothorac Surg 21:711–714

Hurni M, Corno AF, Tucker OP, Payot M, Sekarski N, Cotting J, Bernath MA, von Segesser LK (2000) Venpro: a new pulmonary valved conduit. Thorac Cardiovasc Surg 48(Suppl I):120

Ilbawi MN, Idriss FS, Muster AJ, Wessel HU, Paul MH, DeLeon SY (1981) Tetralogy of Fallot with absent pulmonary valve. Should valve insertion be part of the intracardiac repair? J Thorac Cardiovasc Surg 81:906–915

Karl TR, Musumeci F, de Leval MR, Pincott JR, Taylor JFN, Stark J (1986) Surgical treatment of absent pulmonary valve syndrome. J Thorac Cardiovasc Surg 91:590–597

Lakier JB, Stanger P, Heymann MA, Hoffman JIE, Rudolph AM (1974) Tetralogy of Fallot with absent pulmonary valve. Natural history and hemodynamic considerations. Circulation 50:167–175

Litwin SB, Rosenthal A, Fellows K (1973) Surgical management of young infants with tetralogy of Fallot, absence of the pulmonary valve, and respiratory distress. J Thorac Cardiovasc Surg 65:552–558

Milanesi O, Talenti E, Pellegrino PA, Thiene G (1984) Abnormal pulmonary artery branching in tetralogy of Fallot with "absent" pulmonary valve. Int J Cardiol 6:375–380

Moon-Grady AJ, Tacy TA, Brook MM, Hanley FL, Silverman NH (2002) Value of clinical and echocardiographic features in predicting outcome in the fetus, infant and child with tetralogy of Fallot with absent pulmonary valve complex. Am J Cardiol 89:1280–1285

Rao PS, Lawrie GM (1983) Absent pulmonary valve syndrome: surgical correction with pulmonary arterioplasty. Br Heart J 50:586–589

Snir E, de Leval MR, Elliott MJ, Stark J (1991) Current surgical technique to repair Fallot's tetralogy with absent pulmonary valve syndrome. Ann Thorac Surg 51:979

Stellin G, Jonas RA, Goh TH, Brawn WJ, Venables AW, Mee RBB (1983) Surgical treatment of absent pulmonary valve syndrome in infants: relief of bronchial obstruction. Ann Thorac Surg 36:468–475

Incidence

Pulmonary stenosis is the 2nd most common congenital heart defect, accounting for 9% of all congenital heart diseases. Among all congenital heart malformations, 50% include pulmonary stenosis as a component of the defect. Pulmonary stenosis is more frequent in females.

Morphology

The pulmonary valve leaflets may be fused and/or thickened, with an anomalous insertion to the wall of the proximal main pulmonary artery. The valve opening may be eccentric when the valve leaflets are thick. Sometimes the leaflets are immobile, with an annulus variably small. The right and left pulmonary arteries are generally dilated because of the poststenotic jet effect. Right ventricular hypertrophy is proportional to the degree of stenosis. Dynamic infundibular obstruction may be consequence of muscular hypertrophy of the moderator band: this is usually seen in association with membranous ventricular septal defect; however, the septal defect may spontaneously undergo closure, leaving right ventricular outflow obstruction.

Associated anomalies

Atrial septal defect, ventricular septal defect, peripheral pulmonary stenosis.

Peripheral pulmonary stenosis

▌ This is usually mild with no significant ill consequences. It is seen in neonates due to the smallness of the pulmonary arteries in utero since they carry a small portion of the combined cardiac output to the lungs (7% of the combined cardiac output goes to both lungs). Only about 10–15% will require surgical or balloon dilatation procedures.

▌ In Rubella syndrome the peripheral pulmonary arteries present with bilateral hypoplasia from their origin; it rarely requires therapeutic procedures such as surgery or balloon dilatation.

▌ In Noonan's syndrome peripheral pulmonary stenosis may be seen and older patients with this syndrome may also have cardiomyopathy. This syndrome is associated with lymphedema, webbed neck, dysmorphic features and hypotonia.

▌ In Alagille syndrome diffuse pulmonary stenosis is seen with pulmonary valve stenosis as well as diffuse main and branch pulmonary artery stenosis.

▌ Patients with William's syndrome develop supravalvar pulmonary and aortic stenosis with or without coarctation of the aorta and renal artery stenosis.

Pathophysiology

The right ventricular pressure increases to overcome the stenosis of the pulmonary valve, with an increase in cardiac output due to effort. The extent of stenosis is exaggerated resulting in higher right ventricular pressure until the right ventricular muscles become unable to longer generate enough pressure to overcome the stenosis, resulting in right ventricular failure. The right ventricular hypertrophy and hypertension will result in right ventricular dilatation, leading to left ventricular dysfunction by shifting the interventricular septum and therefore reducing the left ventricular filling.

■ Diagnosis

■ **Clinical pattern:** patients are generally asymptomatic; on auscultation the first heart sound is normal followed by an ejection click; the shorter the distance from S1 to the click, the more severe is the pulmonary stenosis; early systolic click is noted in all cases of pulmonary stenosis except those with dysplasia of the pulmonary valve; absence of a click makes the diagnosis questionable; the murmur is ejection in type, typically harsh and usually 4/6 in intensity or more; the later the peaking of the ejection systolic murmur, the worse is the pulmonary stenosis; the second heart sound is typically widely split and the wider the split the greater the stenosis; a soft P_2 secondary to decreased PA pressure due to severe stenosis may be noted.

■ **Electrocardiogram:** right ventricular hypertrophy with right axis deviation; right atrial enlargement in severe cases.

■ **Chest X-ray:** generally normal heart size; in critical pulmonary stenosis there is an increase in heart size; severe pulmonary stenosis results in decreased pulmonary blood flow, with right-to-left shunting at the level of the patent foramen ovale; mild to moderate pulmonary stenosis is associated with dilatation of the main pulmonary artery and left pulmonary artery.

■ **Echocardiogram:** diagnostic in all cases (Fig. 1.9.1); typically the maximum instanta-

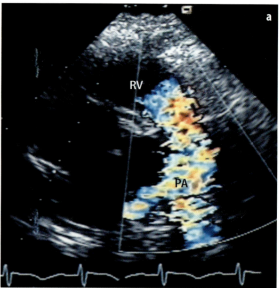

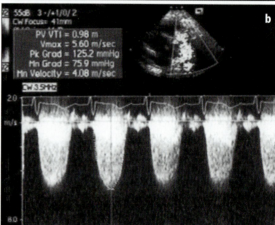

Fig. 1.9.1. Pulmonary valve stenosis: echocardiography. **a** parasternal short axis view showing the turbulence by Doppler color flow through the stenotic pulmonary valve (*PA* pulmonary artery, *RV* right ventricle) (photograph courtesy of Dr. Nicole Sekarski), **b** parasternal short axis view, showing the pressure gradient through the stenotic pulmonary valve measured by Doppler flow (photograph courtesy of Dr. Nicole Sekarski)

neous pressure gradient Doppler is 20–30% more than the peak-to-peak gradient measured at the catheterization laboratory; when planning for balloon dilatation of pulmonary stenosis, the nature of the valve leaflets has to be studied by echocardiography and the pulmonary valve annulus measured to determine the size of the balloon to be used.

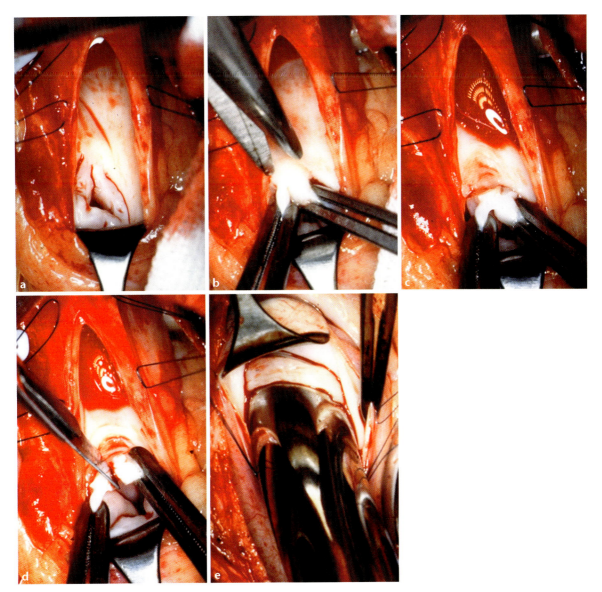

Fig. 1.9.2. Pulmonary valve stenosis: surgery. **a** exposure of a stenotic three-leaflet pulmonary valve through a longitudinal incision on the anterior aspect of the main pulmonary artery, **b** two of the leaflets, controlled with forceps, are separated from their anomalous insertion to the arterial wall by scissors, **c** result obtained in terms of length of the leaflets corresponding to the commissura, separated from the anomalous insertion to the arterial wall, **d** the commissural fusion between the two leaflets, separated from the anomalous insertion to the arterial wall, is now incised with a knife, **e** the diameter of the obtained opening is measured with Hegar dilators and compared with the normal size for age and body weight

▮ **Cardiac catheterization:** all patients with isolated pulmonary valve stenosis with pressure gradients of more than 40–50 mmHg should be catheterized to perform balloon dilatation of the pulmonic valve, unless the pulmonary valve is severely dysplastic with a small annulus.

▮ Indications for surgical treatment

▮ Mild pulmonary valve stenosis (pressure gradient of less than 25 mmHg): therapeutic intervention is not required; SBE prophylaxis is not indicated.

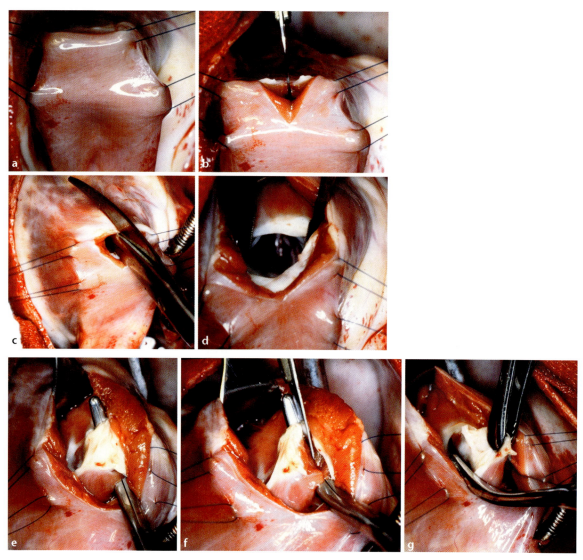

Fig. 1.9.3. Pulmonary valve stenosis with severe subvalvular obstruction: surgery. **a** exposure for a longitudinal right ventriculotomy with two pairs of parallel stay sutures, **b** short longitudinal right ventriculotomy with a knife, **c** after intracardiac inspection, extension of the longitudinal right ventriculotomy with scissors, **d** exposure by opened forceps of the infundibular obstruction, with evident fibrosis of the endocardium, **e** exposure by a surgical instrument of a fibro-muscular trabecula responsible for part of the infundibular obstruction, **f** incision of the fibro-muscular trabecula responsible for part of the infundibular obstruction, **g** resection with scissors of the incised fibro-muscular trabecula, controlled by forceps

▮ Moderate to severe pulmonary stenosis (pressure gradient of 26–49 mmHg): cardiac catheterization should be performed to balloon dilate the stenotic pulmonary valve; results of balloon dilatation is better when the pulmonary stenosis is due to fusion of commissure rather than when the pulmonary valve is dysplastic.

▮ Severe pulmonary stenosis (pressure gradient of 50–79 mmHg): with cyanosis due to right-to-left shunting at the atrial level prostaglandin will be necessary and balloon dilatation of the pulmonary valve may result in relief of much of the pressure gradient across the pulmonary valve.

Suicide right ventricle (severe right ventricular contractility failure) could be seen in patients after balloon dilatation of the pulmonary valve due to right ventricular outflow tract obstruction secondary to musculature hypertrophy of the right ventricular outflow tract. This is also noted post surgical relief and particularly in patients with an initial right ventricular pressure of more than 100 mmHg. It is rare nowadays to see patients with this kind of pressure in the right ventricle as they are treated early enough.

■ Critical pulmonary stenosis (ductus-dependent pulmonary blood flow): with near atresia of the pulmonic valve, the right ventricle is hypertrophied yet with a very small cavity, as in pulmonary atresia with intact ventricular septum (see chapter "Pulmonary atresia with intact ventricular septum").

■ Surgical treatment

Nowadays the need for surgical treatment of isolated pulmonary valve stenosis is very rare.

In the case of pulmonary valve stenosis with associated cardiac defects, the surgical treatment consists in pulmonary valvotomy on cardiopulmonary bypass (Fig. 1.9.2): through a longitudinal incision on the anterior aspect of the main pulmonary artery, the pulmonary valve is exposed; the leaflets are separated from their anomalous insertion to the arterial wall, the commissural fusions are incised and the diameter of the obtained opening is measured with Hegar dilators and compared with the normal size for age and body weight.

In the presence of a dysplastic pulmonary valve, a pulmonary valvectomy (excision of the pulmonary valve) can be performed, leaving a pulmonary valve regurgitation.

In the presence of a hypoplastic pulmonary valve annulus, a transannular incision is performed and the annulus is enlarged with a transannular patch, generally of autologous or heterologous pericardium.

If pulmonary valve stenosis is accompanied by severe subvalvular obstruction, infundibular resection through a right ventriculotomy may be required (Fig. 1.9.3).

■ Potential complications

Residual or recurrent pulmonary valve stenosis, pulmonary valve regurgitation.

■ References

Brock RC (1948) Pulmonary valvotomy for the relief of congenital pulmonary stenosis. Br Med J 1:1121

Campbell M (1954) Simple pulmonary stenosis. Br Heart J 16:273

Cheng TO (2002) Acute pulmonary edema complicating percutaneous balloon valvuloplasty for pulmonic stenosis. J Cardiothorac Vasc Anesth 16:391

Corno AF, von Segesser LK (1999) Is hypothermia necessary in pediatric cardiac surgery? Eur J Cardiothorac Surg 15:110–111

Danilowicz D, Hoffman JIE, Rudolph AM (1975) Serial studies of pulmonary stenosis in infancy and childhood. Br Heart J 37:808–818

Fyler DC, Buckley LP, Hellenbrand WE, Cohn HE (1980) Report of the New England Regional Infant Care Program. Pediatrics 65(Suppl):375–461

Gikonyo BM, Lucas RV, Edwards JE (1978) Anatomic features of congenital pulmonary valvar stenosis. Pediatr Cardiol 8:109–115

Guntheroth WG (2002) Causes and effects of poststenotic dilatation of the pulmonary trunk. Am J Cardiol 89:774–776

Hoffman JIE, Kaplan S (2002) The incidence of congenital heart disease. J Am Coll Cardiol 39:1890–1900

Kan JS, White RI, Mitchell SE, Gardner TJ (1983) Percutaneous balloon valvuloplasty: a new method for treating congenital pulmonary and valve stenosis. N Engl J Med 370:540–542

Lam J, Corno AF, Oorthuys HKE, Marcelletti C (1983) Unusual association of congenital heart disease in Noonan's syndrome. Pediatr Cardiol 3:23–26

Latson LA (2001) Critical pulmonary stenosis. J Interv Cardiol 14:345–350

Marino B, Corno AF, Carotti A, Pasquini L, Giannico S, Guccione P, Bevilacqua M, De Simone G, Marcelletti C (1990) Pediatric cardiac surgery guided by echocardiography. Scand J Thorac Cardiovasc Surg 24:197–201

McGoon DC, Kirklin JW (1958) Pulmonic stenosis with intact ventricular septum. Treatment utilizing extracorporeal circulation. Circulation 17:180

Mitchell SC, Korones SB, Berendes HW (1971) Congenital heart disease in 56,109 births. Incidence and natural history. Circulation 43:323

Noonan JA, Ehmke DA (1963) Associated non-cardiac malformations in children with congenital heart disease. J Pediatr 63:468–470

Sellors TH (1948) Surgery of pulmonary stenosis: a case in which the pulmonary valve was successfully divided. Lancet 1:988–989

Vancini M, Roberts KD, Silove MD, Singh SP (1980) Surgical treatment of congenital pulmonary valve stenosis due to dysplastic leaflets and a small valve annulus. J Thorac Cardiovasc Surg 79:464–468

CHAPTER 1.10 Pulmonary atresia with intact ventricular septum

Incidence

This is the 13th most common congenital heart disease (1.7% of all congenital heart defects). It occurs in 0.08/1000 live births.

Morphology

The pulmonary valve annulus is usually small but not hypoplastic. The pulmonary valve leaflets are well formed but fused. The main pulmonary artery is small but is rarely atretic as seen with pulmonary atresia and ventricular septal defect. The patent ductus arteriosus is usually small because it carries blood from the aorta to the pulmonary arteries in utero and not the other way around as is normal; therefore, much less blood travels through the patent ductus arteriosus in utero.

The right ventricle might be of several types:
- Type I: tripartite
- Type II: bipartite (atretic body)
- Type III: unipartite (atretic body and infundibulum).

Tricuspid valve might be deformed and stenotic.

Associated anomalies

Other congenital heart defects are rarely associated. Right aortic arch is not known to occur in pulmonary atresia with intact ventricular septum. The origin and distribution of the coronary arteries may exhibit the

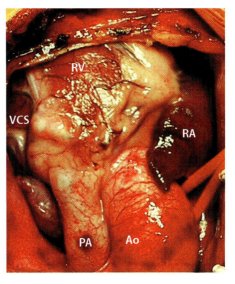

Fig. 1.10.1. Pulmonary atresia with intact ventricular septum. Intra-operative photograph, showing very dilated ventriculo-coronary sinusoids in correspondence of the right ventricular outflow tract (*Ao* aorta, *VCS* ventriculo-coronary sinusoids, *PA* pulmonary artery, *RA* right atrium, *RV* right ventricle)

same variability as the normal heart, including the presence of coronary artery stenosis. Ventriculo-coronary sinusoids are frequent from the right ventricular cavity to the myocardium and from the myocardium to the coronary arteries (Fig. 1.10.1). Collateral circulation from the descending aorta to pulmonary arteries is rare.

Pathophysiology

Egress of blood determines right ventricular pressure and size. The more egress through the tricuspid valve into the right atrium or from the sinusoids into the coronary arteries, the lower the right ventricular pressure. The more the tricuspid valve regurgitation, the larger the right ventricle and right atrial sizes. The systemic venous return will go from the right atrium predominantly through a patent foramen ovale to the left atrium causing cyanosis. The patent foramen ovale is frequently restrictive, but the pressure gradient is rarely more than 2–3 mmHg.

The pulmonary circulation is ductus dependent.

Intrinsic to the presence of ventriculo-coronary sinusoids is the pathophysiologic pattern of right ventricular dependent coronary artery circulation.

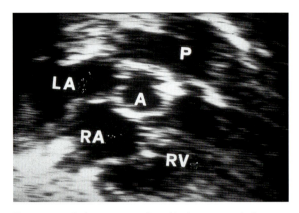

Fig. 1.10.2. Pulmonary atresia with intact ventricular septum: echocardiography (*A* aorta, *LA* left atrium, *P* pulmonary artery, *RA* right atrium, *RV* right ventricle) (photograph courtesy of Dr. Bruno Marino)

▮ Diagnosis

▮ **Clinical pattern:** at birth the ductus arteriosus provides pulmonary blood flow and there may or may not be cyanosis evident in the immediate neonatal period; as the ductus arteriosus closes, there will be less pulmonary blood flow causing cyanosis; physical findings will be consistent with cyanosis, patent ductus arteriosus murmur, a systolic murmur secondary to tricuspid valve regurgitation and a single second heart sound.

▮ **Electrocardiogram:** frontal QRS axis from +30° to +90°, small right ventricular forces; right atrial enlargement is common; ST-T wave abnormalities are quite common, and they may progress.

▮ **Chest X-ray:** mild to moderate cardiac enlargement, reduced lung vascularization.

▮ **Echocardiogram:** pulmonary blood flow is supplied through the patent ductus arteriosus; the valve leaflets are fused and there is variable hypoplasia of the right ventricle (Fig. 1.10.2); the main pulmonary artery tends to be well developed; the diameter of the tricuspid regurgitation obtained by color Doppler and the size of the right atrium are good indicators of the severity of tricuspid

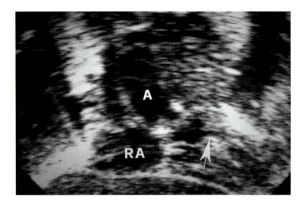

Fig. 1.10.3. Pulmonary atresia with intact ventricular septum: echocardiography showing right ventricle to coronary arteries sinusoids (white arrow) (*A* aorta, *RA* right atrium) (photograph courtesy of Dr. Bruno Marino)

valve regurgitation; the right ventricular size generally corresponds with the dimension of the tricuspid annulus; sometimes it is possible to identify right ventricle to coronary arteries sinusoids (Fig. 1.10.3); it is important to distinguish anatomic from functional pulmonary atresia.

▮ **Cardiac catheterization:** indicated in the presence of a small-sized, hypertensive right ventricular cavity (Figs. 1.10.4 and 1.10.5); Rashkind atrial septostomy may be needed as well as the assessment of right ventricle to coronary arteries sinusoids.

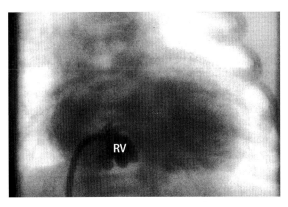

Fig. 1.10.4. Pulmonary atresia with intact ventricular septum: angiography. Antero-posterior view, with contrast injection showing the diminutive size of the right ventricular cavity (*RV* right ventricle)

▋ Indications for surgical treatment

Prostaglandin E infusion is utilized to maintain the ductus arteriosus open, to provide pulmonary blood flow.

▋ Surgical treatment

The right ventricular size and function dictate the possibility of surgical treatment with biventricular or univentricular type of repair, or one and half ventricular repair.

Surgical pulmonary valvotomy (generally on cardiopulmonary bypass) with or without systemic-to-pulmonary arterial shunt depending upon the right ventricular size. If the right ventricle is small, a systemic-to-pulmonary arterial shunt is necessary to provide pulmonary blood flow until antegrade flow through the pulmonary valve is adequate. However, if the pulmonary arteries are not small, then pulmonary valvotomy alone may be adequate, with or without a post-operative period with maintained prostaglandin E infusion.

Decompression of the right ventricle by pulmonary valvotomy (or by tricuspid valve avulsion) may cause reversal of flow in the coronary arteries to sinusoids, leading to poor myocardial perfusion. This is especially true in the presence of coronary artery ste-

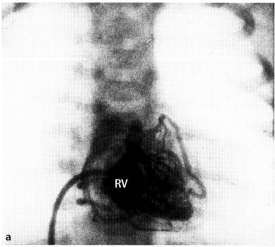

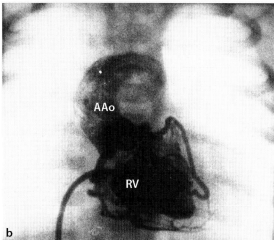

Fig. 1.10.5. Pulmonary atresia with intact ventricular septum: angiography. **a** antero-posterior view, with contrast injection showing the diminutive size of the right ventricular cavity and the numerous right ventricle to coronary arteries sinusoids (*RV* right ventricle), **b** subsequent imaging showing the opacification of the ascending aorta by the right ventricle to coronary arteries sinusoids (*AAo* ascending aorta, *RV* right ventricle)

nosis. Therefore, right ventricular decompression should not be performed if coronary artery stenoses are noted with sinusoids.

In patients with small pulmonary arteries treated with a systemic-to-pulmonary artery shunt, if the right ventricle continues to be small and inadequate, then a cavo-pulmonary connection may be required.

Patients with severe right ventricle to coronary arteries sinusoids may require cardiac transplantation. Sinusoids are typically not present in patients with severe tricuspid insufficiency and a normal right ventricular size. In patients with significant tricuspid valve regurgitation and low right ventricular pressure, pulmonary valvotomy may not result in effective forward flow through the right ventricle because of the tricuspid valve regurgitation.

∎ Potential complications

Inadequate pulmonary blood flow, poor myocardial perfusion, myocardial infarction, residual tricuspid valve regurgitation, right heart failure.

∎ References

Albanese SB, Carotti A, Toscano A, Marino B, di Donato RM (2002) Pulmonary atresia with intact ventricular septum and systemic-pulmonary collateral arteries. Ann Thorac Surg 73:1322–1324

Amodeo A, Keeton BR, Sutherland GR, Monro JL (1991) Pulmonary atresia with intact ventricular septum: is neonatal repair advisable? Eur J Cardiothorac Surg 5:17

Billingsley AM, Laks H, Boyce SW, George BL, Santulli T, Williams RG (1989) Definitive repair in patients with pulmonary atresia and intact ventricular septum. J Thorac Cardiovasc Surg 97:746–754

Bull C, de Leval MR, Mercanti C, Macartney FJ, Anderson RH (1982) Pulmonary atresia and intact ventricular septum: a revised classification. Circulation 66:266–272

Cheung YF, Leung MP, Chau AK (2002) Usefulness of laser-assisted valvotomy with balloon valvoplasty for pulmonary atresia with intact ventricular septum. Am J Cardiol 15:438–442

Corno AF, Mazzera E, Marino B, Parisi F, Marcelletti C (1986) Simultaneous patency of ductus arteriosus and surgical shunt in pulmonary atresia with intact ventricular septum. A cause of acute myocardial failure? Scand J Thorac Cardiovasc Surg 20:123–127

Corno AF, Giannico S, Marino B, Parisi F, Marcelletti C (1988) Atresia polmonare con setto interventricolare intatto: risultati a distanza. Cardiol 33(Suppl II):18

Corno AF, Mazzera E, Marino B, Picardo S, Marcelletti C (1989) Bidirectional cavopulmonary anastomosis. J Am Coll Cardiol 13:74A

Corno AF, Giannico S (1993) Echo evaluation of total extracardiac right heart bypass. G Ital Ecogr Cardiovasc 3:1

Corno AF, Bertucci C, Ranucci M, Rosti L (1994) Bidirectional superior vena cava to pulmonary artery anastomosis. Int Soc Cardiothorac Surg, 4th World Congr, Abstracts, p 150

Corno AF (1996) Considerations on the cavopulmonary connection. Am Coll Cardiol Curr J Rev 5:38

Corno AF, Da Cruz E, Lal AB, Milella L, Wilson N (1998) "Controlled reoxygenation" for cyanotic patients. In: Imai Y, Momma K (eds) Proceedings of 2nd World Congress of PCCS. Futura Publishing Co, Armonk, NY, pp 1127–1129

Corno AF, Hurni M, Payot M, von Segesser LK (1999) Modified Blalock-Taussig shunt with compensatory properties. Ann Thorac Surg 67:269–270

Corno AF, von Segesser LK (1999) Is hypothermia necessary in pediatric cardiac surgery? Eur J Cardiothorac Surg 15:110–111

Corno AF (2000) Surgery for congenital heart disease. Curr Opinion Cardiol 15:238–243

Daubeney PE, Delany DJ, Anderson RH, Sandor GG, Slavik Z, Keeton BR, Webber SA (2002) Pulmonary atresia with intact ventricular septum: range of morphology in a population-based study. J Am Coll Cardiol 15:1670–1679

De Leval MR, Bull C, Stark J, Anderson RH, Taylor JFN, Macartney FJ (1982) Pulmonary atresia and intact ventricular septum: surgical management based on a revised classification. Circulation 66:272–280

Freedom RM, Harrington DP (1974) Contributions of intramyocardial sinusoids in pulmonary atresia and intact ventricular septum to a right-sided circular shunt. Br Heart J 36:1061

Freedom RM (1983) The morphological variations of pulmonary atresia with intact ventricular septum: guidelines for surgical intervention. Pediatr Cardiol 4:183–188

Fyler DC, Buckley LP, Hellenbrand WE, Cohn HE (1980) Report of the New England Regional Infant Care Program. Pediatrics 65(Suppl):375–461

Gagliardi MG, Marino B, Papa M, Corno AF, Squitieri C, Marcelletti C (1989) Atresia polmonare a setto integro: indicazioni al trattamento chirurgico neonatale guidato dall'ecocardiografia bidimensionale e Doppler. G Ital Cardiol 19:315–318

Giannico S, Corno AF, Nava S, Marino B, Guccione P, Marcelletti C (1989) Inferior vena cava to pulmonary artery extracardiac conduit: echo-Doppler patterns of systemic venous flow. J Am Soc Echocard 2:218

Giannico S, Corno AF, Marino B, Cicini MP, Gagliardi MG, Amodeo A, Picardo S, Marcelletti C (1992) Total extracardiac right heart bypass. Circulation 86(Suppl 2):110–117

Grabitz RG, Joffres MR, Collins-Nakai RL (1988) Congenital heart disease: incidence in the first year of life. The Alberta heritage pediatric cardiology program. Am J Epidemiol 128:381–388

Hoffman JIE, Kaplan S (2002) The incidence of congenital heart disease. J Am Coll Cardiol 39:1890–1900

Marino B, Corno AF, Pasquini L, Guccione P, Carta MG, Ballerini L, De Simone G, Marcelletti C (1987) Indication for systemic-pulmonary artery shunts guided by two-dimensional and Doppler echocardiography: criteria for patient selection. Ann Thorac Surg 44:495–498

Marino B, Giannico S, Pasquini L, Corno AF, Picardo S (1988) Balloon-occlusion of the carotid artery for the angiographic visualization of Blalock-Taussig shunts and pulmonary arteries. Chest 94:267–269

Mazzera E, Corno AF, Picardo S, Di Donato RM, Marino B, Costa D, Marcelletti C (1989) Bidirectional cavopulmonary shunts: clinical applications as staged or definitive palliation. Ann Thorac Surg 47:415–420

Marcelletti C, Corno AF, Giannico S, Marino B (1990) Inferior vena cava to pulmonary artery extracardiac conduit: a new form of right heart bypass. J Thorac Cardiovasc Surg 100:228–232

Minich LL, Tani LY, Ritter S, Williams RV, Shaddy RE, Hawkins JA (2000) Usefulness of the preoperative tricuspid/mitral valve ratio for predicting outcome in pulmonary atresia with intact ventricular septum. Am J Cardiol 85:1325–1328

Olley PM, Coceani F, Bodach E (1976) E-type prostaglandins: a new emergency therapy for certain cyanotic congenital heart malformations. Circulations 53:728–731

Powell AJ, Mayer JE, Lang P, Lock JE (2000) Outcome in infants with pulmonary atresia, intact ventricular septum and right ventricle-dependent coronary circulation. Am J Cardiol 86:1272–1274

Qureshi SA (2001) Collaborative approach in the management of pulmonary atresia with intact ventricular septum. J Interv Cardiol 14:377–384

Sano S, Ishino K, Kawada M, Fujisawa E, Kamada M, Ohtsuki S (2000) Staged biventricular repair of pulmonary atresia or stenosis with intact ventricular septum. Ann Thorac Surg 70:1501–1506

Schire V, Sutin GL, Barnard CN (1961) Organic and functional pulmonary atresia with intact ventricular septum. Am J Cardiol 8:100–108

Shimpo H, Hayakawa H, Miyake Y, Takabayashi S, Yada I (2000) Strategy for pulmonary atresia and intact ventricular septum. Ann Thorac Surg 70:287–289

Takayama H, Sekiguchi A, Chikada M (2001) Pulmonary atresia with intact ventricular septum: long-term results of "one and a half ventricular repair". Updated in 2001. Ann Thorac Surg 72:2178–2179

Tulzer G, Arzt W, Franklin RC, Loughna PV, Mair R, Gardiner HM (2002) Fetal pulmonary valvuloplasty for critical pulmonary stenosis or atresia with intact septum. Lancet 360:1567–1568

Weber HS (2002) Initial and late results after catheter intervention for neonatal critical pulmonary valve stenosis and atresia with intact ventricular septum: a technique in continual evolution. Catheter Cardiovasc Interv 56:394–399

Zuberbuhler JR, Anderson RH (1979) Morphological variations in pulmonary atresia with intact ventricular septum. Br Heart J 41:281

CHAPTER 1.11 Ebstein's anomaly

Incidence

Ebstein's anomaly is the 18th most common congenital heart defect (1% of all congenital heart defects). It occurs in 0.3–0.8% of all congenital heart diseases in the first year of life, 1:20000–50000 live births. There is equal male to female occurrence.

Morphology

There are five anatomic characteristics of the Ebstein's anomaly (Fig. 1.11.1), relevant to the surgical management of the condition:

- Displacement of the septal and posterior leaflets of the tricuspid valve towards the apex of the right ventricle, with adherence to the myocardium.
- Anterior leaflet attached to the appropriate level of the tricuspid valve annulus, however, redundant, larger than normal and with multiple fenestrations and chordal attachments to the ventricular wall.
- The segment of the right ventricle from the level of the true tricuspid annulus to the level of attachment of the septal and posterior leaflets unusually thin and dysplastic, and described as "atrialized"; tricuspid annulus and right atrium extremely dilated.
- Cavity of the right ventricle, beyond the atrialized portion, reduced in size, usually with lack of an inlet chamber, and with a small trabecular component.
- Infundibulum often obstructed by the redundant tissue of the anterior leaflet as well as by the chordal attachments of the anterior leaflet to the infundibulum.

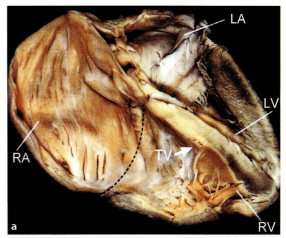
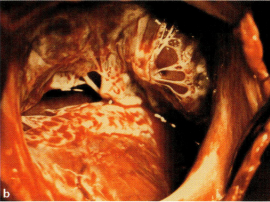

Fig. 1.11.1. Ebstein's anomaly: morphology. **a** pathology specimen (*LA* left atrium, *LV* left ventricle, *RA* right atrium, *RV* right ventricle, *TV* tricuspid valve (photograph courtesy of Dr. Enrico Chiappa), **b** intra-operative photograph from a right atriotomy (photograph courtesy of Dr. Sylvain Chauvaud)

In addition, there are four clinical variants (Carpentier classification) with progressively increasing severity:

- Type A: the volume of the true right ventricle is adequate;

- Type B: the volume of the right ventricle is small, and there is a large atrialized portion of the right ventricle;
- Type C: the volume of the right ventricle is small, with right ventricular outflow tract obstruction;
- Type D: there is almost complete atrialization of the right ventricle with the exception of a small infundibular component, and the only communication between the atrialized ventricle and the infundibulum is through the antero-septal commissura of the tricuspid valve.

￭ Associated anomalies

The most common associated anomaly is atrial septal defect, occurring in about 50% of cases.

There is a variable degree of right ventricular outflow tract obstruction. A Wolff-Parkinson-White type of accessory pathway, often with associated pre-excitation, is present in about 10% of cases. In symptomatic neonates, survival is dependent on the presence of a patent ductus arteriosus. Rarely, an abnormality of ventriculo-arterial connection or double discordance (atrioventricular and ventriculo-arterial) is associated, atrioventricular septal defect, ventricular septal defect, tetralogy of Fallot, or aortic coarctation. It can be present in patients with Down syndrome, Marfan's syndrome, Ulrich-Noonan syndrome and Cornelia de Lange syndrome.

￭ Pathophysiology

The right atrium is dilated secondary to tricuspid valve anomalies and tricuspid insufficiency.

The anterior tricuspid valve leaflet forms a large sail-like structure with or without fenestrations and with or without blood flow obstruction; when there is no fenestration of the tricuspid valve leaflet, the result is tricuspid valve stenosis.

In severe cases, the inferior right ventricular wall is thin and void of muscle cells, thus, forming an aneurysmal structure. The right ventricle is dilated and the interventricular septum bulges leftward: this may impair left ventricular function. The patent foramen ovale is almost always patent, sometimes associated with an ostium secundum atrial septal defect. The shunt at the atrial level can be left-to-right, right-to-left or bidirectional, accordingly with the presence and degree of right atrial hypertension due to right heart failure.

Patients with Ebstein's malformation are prone to arrhythmias because:
- The right atrium is dilated resulting in stretching and fibrosis which would lead to arrhythmias.
- Poor fibrous development of the atrioventricular ring causing bypass tracts from the atria to the ventricles and resulting in Wolf-Parkinson-White syndrome (WPW): there may be numerous tracts in as many as 20–25% of patients.
- Poor fibrous encasement of the atrioventricular node and bundle of His will cause atrioventricular re-entry tachycardia.
- Ventricular arrhythmias from the stretched, fibrotic and dysplastic tissue of the right ventricle.

Sudden death is encountered in 3–10% of patients, secondary to supraventricular tachycardia leading to ventricular tachycardia or fast conduction of atrial fibrillation or flutter.

￭ Diagnosis

￭ **Natural history:** Mortality in children presenting in the neonatal period is 30–50%. Mortality at all ages is 12.5%. Mortality is higher with severe right atrial enlargement, large atrialized right ventricular portion, distally tethered tricuspid valve leaflet and right ventricular dysplasia. Mortality rate is higher in patients with other associated congenital heart diseases, when presentation is in infancy and with severe cyanosis or congestive heart failure.

When Ebstein's malformation presents in the neonatal period, it may be due to severe tricuspid valve regurgitation with severely dilated right atrium, similar to pulmonary atresia with intact ventricular septum, or similar to tricuspid atresia due to obstruction of the tricuspid valve.

On the other hand, if the Ebstein's malformation is mild and the right atrium does not dilate significantly soon after birth due to a drop in the pulmonary vascular resistance, the clinical situation may improve.

▌ **Clinical pattern:** patients may present with cyanosis, syncope, congestive heart failure, palpitation, sudden death and/or paradoxical embolization; the severity of the symptoms do not necessarily correlate with the severity of the pathological changes of the tricuspid valve; on examination cyanosis and clubbing are common; there is sometimes a deformed chest wall secondary to cardiomegaly; the precordium is usually quite despite cardiomegaly; systolic thrill is sometimes present; there are normal neck veins even with severe tricuspid regurgitation, secondary to a large compliant right atrium; auscultation: the most striking finding is triple or quadruple rhythm secondary to added sounds, which may result from a split S_1 due to the delay in tricuspid valve closure; S_2 is widely and persistently split secondary to right bundle branch block and delayed right ventricular semilunar valve closure; also, ventricular filling sounds are present.

▌ **Electrocardiogram:** PR interval is prolonged in 16–42% of cases; right axis deviation, right atrial enlargement and right bundle branch block; decrease in the R amplitude in V_1 through V_4; absent Q wave in V_6 due to ventricular displacement secondary to a dilated right atrium; complete or incomplete right bundle branch block is seen in 77–94% of cases; 4–26% of patients also have Wolf-Parkinson-White syndrome, usually B type.

▌ **Chest X-ray:** the size of the heart varies anywhere from normal to severe cardiomegaly; right atrial enlargement is the main cause of cardiomegaly and this may cause displacement of the left ventricle posteriorly; pulmonary blood flow is decreased or within normal limits.

▌ **Echocardiogram:** the morphology and the functional severity can be assessed by the following observations:
▌ presence and amount of right-to-left shunt at the atrial level (Fig. 1.11.2),
▌ degree of tricuspid regurgitation (width of jet at origin and whether it goes to the hepatic veins) (Fig. 1.11.3),
▌ right atrial and ventricular size (Fig. 1.11.4) and function,
▌ left ventricular function.

In addition, echocardiography can assess the potential response to surgery by assessing the following anatomy:
▌ displacement of septal leaflet (Fig. 1.11.4),
▌ tethering of anterior leaflet,
▌ fenestration of anterior leaflet,
▌ leaflet dysplasia,
▌ right ventricular enlargement, aneurysm of right ventricular outflow tract.

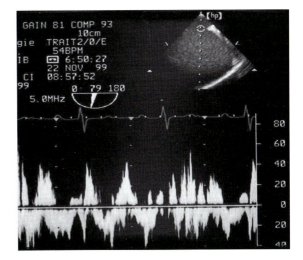

Fig. 1.11.2. Ebstein's anomaly: echocardiography. Transesophageal Doppler echocardiography showing bi-directional shunt through the atrial septal defect (photograph courtesy of Dr. Pierre-Guy Chassot)

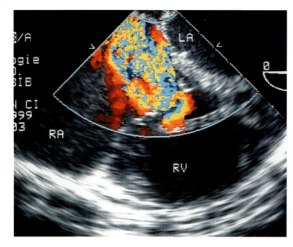

Fig. 1.11.3. Ebstein's anomaly: echocardiography. Transesophageal color Doppler echocardiography showing the tricuspid valve regurgitation (*LA* left atrium, *RA* right atrium, *RV* right ventricle) (photograph courtesy of Dr. Pierre-Guy Chassot)

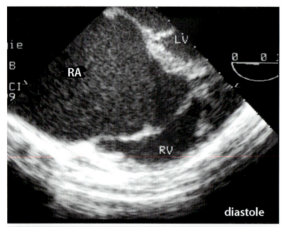

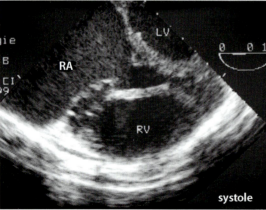

Fig. 1.11.4. Ebstein's anomaly: echocardiography. Transesophageal echocardiography showing the size of the right atrium and ventricle, and the displacement of the anterior leaflet of the tricuspid valve (*LV* left ventricle, *RA* right atrium, *RV* right ventricle) (photograph courtesy of Dr. Pierre-Guy Chassot)

■ **Cardiac catheterization:** cardiac catheterization is risky as it may lead to arrhythmia; therefore,
– it should be done cautiously;
– indicated only to rule out associated complex conditions.

■ Indications for surgical treatment

In symptomatic neonates with Ebstein's anomaly, surgery is indicated because of severe tricuspid valve regurgitation with severely dilated right atrium and right-to-left shunt at the atrial level, with reduced pulmonary blood flow, similar to pulmonary atresia with intact ventricular septum. In children surgery is indicated because of cyanosis and heart failure. In adults the main symptoms can be cyanosis, congestive heart failure and arrhythmias.

■ Surgical treatment (on cardiopulmonary bypass)

When repairing Ebstein's anomaly, it is important to have intra-operative transesophageal echocardiography to assess the result of the surgical procedure.

The surgical repair includes:
■ Closure of the atrial septal defect.
■ Plication of the atrialized portion of the right ventricle (Fig. 1.11.5).
■ Repair of the tricuspid valve by replacing the anterior leaflet.

Tricuspid valve replacement is very rarely required.

In patients with reduced size or function of the right ventricle, a one-and-half ventricular repair is performed, with end-to-side anastomosis of the superior vena cava to the right pulmonary artery in addition to the intra-cardiac repair, in order to reduce the volume overload of the small/malfunctioning right ventricle (Fig. 1.11.6). As an exception a total cavo-pulmonary connection (univentricular repair) is required for patients with

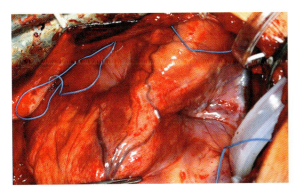

Fig. 1.11.5. Ebstein's anomaly. Intra-operative photograph showing the external appearance of the plication of the atrialized portion of the right ventricle

extremely small or malfunctioning right ventricle.

Pre-operative electro-physiology for by-pass pathways is necessary in order to perform intra-operative ablation.

When ventricular pacing is required, it should be done through epicardial leads rather intravenously, since the tricuspid valve's function is already compromised.

▮ Potential complications

Residual or recurrent atrial septal defect, residual or recurrent (or surgically induced) tricuspid valve stenosis or insufficiency, complete atrioventricular block, right coronary artery obstruction during the process of plication, right ventricular dysfunction, left ventricular dysfunction.

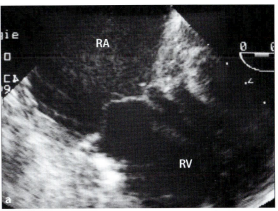

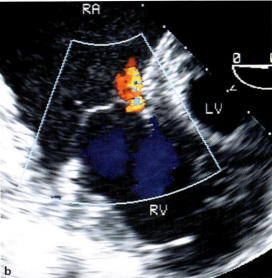

Fig. 1.11.6. Ebstein's anomaly: echocardiography. Post-operative transesophageal echocardiography after reconstruction of the tricuspid valve, plication of the atrialized portion of the right ventricle and end-to-side superior vena cava to right pulmonary artery anastomosis: **a** repositioning of the anterior leaflet of the tricuspid valve (see Fig. 1.11.4 with the pre-operative echocardiography of the same patient), **b** reduced degree of the tricuspid valve (see Fig. 1.11.3 with the pre-operative echocardiography of the same patient) (photographs courtesy of Dr. Pierre-Guy Chassot)

■ References

Barnard CN, Schire V (1963) Surgical correction of Ebstein's malformation with a prosthetic tricuspid valve. Surgery 54:302

Becker AE, Becker MJ, Edwards JE (1971) Pathologic spectrum of dysplasia of the tricuspid valve. Features in common with Ebstein's malformation. Arch Pathol 91:167–178

Carpentier A, Chauvaud S, Macé L, Relland J, Mihaileanu S, Marino JP, Abry B, Guibourt P (1988) A new reconstructive operation for Ebstein's anomaly of the tricuspid valve. J Thorac Cardiovasc Surg 96:92

Corno AF, Mazzera E, Marino B, Picardo S, Marcelletti C (1989) Bidirectional cavopulmonary anastomosis. J Am Coll Cardiol 13:74A

Corno AF (2000) Surgery for congenital heart disease. Curr Opinion Cardiol 15:238–243

Corno AF, Chassot PG, Payot M, Sekarski N, Tozzi P, von Segesser LK (2002) Ebstein's anomaly: one and half ventricular repair. Swiss Med Weekly 132:485–488

Davtyan HG, Corno AF, Drinkwater DC, George B, Laks H (1986) Valve replacement for congenital heart disease. Circulation 74:II–250

Danielson GK, Driscoll DJ, Mair DD, Warnes CA, Oliver WC (1992) Operative treatment of Ebstein's anomaly. J Thorac Cardiovasc Surg 104: 1195–1202

Di Russo GB, Gaynor JW (1999) Ebstein's anomaly: indications for repair and surgical technique. Semin Thorac Cardiovasc Surg 2:35–50

Fyler DC, Buckley LP, Hellenbrand WE, Cohn HE (1980) Report of the New England Regional Infant Care Program. Pediatrics 65(Suppl):375–461

Gasul BM, Weinberg M, Luan LL, Fell EH, Bicoff J, Steiger Z (1959) Superior vena cava-right main pulmonary artery anastomosis. Surgical correction for patients with Ebstein's anomaly and for congenital hypoplastic right ventricle. JAMA 171:1797–1803

Hardy KL, May IA, Webster CA, Kimball KG (1964) Ebstein's anomaly: a functional concept and successful definitive repair. J Thorac Cardiovasc Surg 48:927

Haworth SG, Shinebourne EA, Miller GAH (1975) Right-to-left interatrial shunting with normal right ventricular pressure. A puzzling haemodynamic picture associated with some rare congenital malformations of the tricuspid valve and right ventricle. Br Heart J 37:386–391

Knott-Craig CJ, Overholt ED, Ward KE, Ringewald JM, Baker SS, Razook JD (2002) Repair of Ebstein's anomaly in the symptomatic neonate: an evolution of technique with 7-year follow-up. Ann Thorac Surg 73:1786–1792

Mazzera E, Corno AF, Picardo S, Di Donato RM, Marino B, Costa D, Marcelletti C (1989) Bidirectional cavopulmonary shunts: clinical applications as staged or definitive palliation. Ann Thorac Surg 47:415–420

Reddy VM, McElhinney DB, Silverman NH, Marianeschi SM, Hanley FL (1998) Partial biventricular repair for complex congenital heart defects: an intermediate option for complicated anatomy or functionally borderline right complex heart. J Thorac Cardiovasc Surg 116:21–27

Sano S, Ishino K, Kawada M, Kasahara S, Kohmoto S, Takeuchi M, Ohtsuki S (2002) Total right ventricular exclusion procedure: an operation for isolated congestive right ventricular failure. J Thorac Cardiovasc Surg 123:640–647

Schire V, Sutin GL, Barnard CN (1961) Organic and functional pulmonary atresia with intact ventricular septum. Am J Cardiol 8:100–108

Watson H (1974) Natural history of Ebstein's anomaly of the tricuspid valve in childhood and adolescence: an international cooperative study of 505 cases. Br Heart J 36:417

Wu Q, Huang Z (2001) Anatomic correction of Ebstein anomaly. J Thorac Cardiovasc Surg 122: 1237–1238

Zuberbuhler JR, Allwork SP, Anderson RH (1979) The spectrum of Ebstein's anomaly of the tricuspid valve. J Thorac Cardiovasc Surg 77:202–211

Patent ductus arteriosus

▌ Incidence

Patent ductus arteriosus is the most common congenital heart defect in neonates. Its elevated incidence is related to the increased survival of premature infants, delayed ductal closure being very frequent in these infants, with an incidence varying from 20% in prematures born after 32 weeks of pregnancy to 60% in those born after 28 weeks of pregnancy. Patent ductus arteriosus accounts for about 10% of congenital heart defects in term neonates, and it ranks the 10th most common congenital heart defect in infants (2.4% of all congenital heart defects). Patent ductus arteriosus is more frequent in females.

▌ Morphology (Fig. 1.12.1)

The ductus arteriosus connects the aortic arch opposite of the left subclavian artery to the left pulmonary artery. Patent ductus arteriosus, when it closes, usually does so beginning from the pulmonary artery end, leaving a diverticulum in the aortic site (Kommerel diverticulum) which eventually closes. The patent ductus arteriosus is connected to the left pulmonary artery even in the presence of right aortic arch. Rarely it connects to the right pulmonary artery. Bilateral patent ductus arteriosus has very rarely been observed.

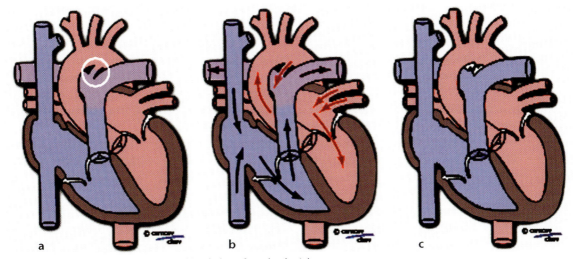

Fig. 1.12.1. Patent ductus arteriosus. **a** Morphology, **b** pathophysiology, **c** surgery

▌ Associated anomalies

Atrial septal defect, atrioventricular septal defect, ventricular septal defect, aortic coarctation, tetralogy of Fallot, transposition of the great arteries and the group of ductus-dependent congenital heart defects: hypoplastic left heart, aortic arch interruption, pulmonary atresia with or without intact ventricular septum.

▌ Pathophysiology

In premature infants the patent ductus arteriosus closes later than it would in term babies. However, if the prematurity is taken into consideration, it closes about the same time. Patent ductus arteriosus closes with high oxygen tension, which explains why at high altitude the patent ductus arteriosus remain patent for a longer time. The etiology of higher incidence of patent ductus arteriosus in maternal rubella infection is not clear but it could be due to tissue changes in the ductus arteriosus similar to those observed in right pulmonary artery and left pulmonary artery branches. Indomethacin if given to the mother at pre-term will cause the patent ductus arteriosus to constrict: this is due to interference with the arachidonic derivative causing lack of prostaglandin. Supplemental oxygen will cause the patent ductus arteriosus to close in full term but not in premature babies. On the other hand, prostaglandin is better at keeping the patent ductus arteriosus open in prematures versus full term babies.

Like all arterial-level shunts, flow occurs during both systole and diastole; the magnitude depends on both the size of the duct and the relative resistance of the pulmonary and systemic circulations.

Due to the left-to-right shunting at the patent ductus arteriosus, the pulmonary venous return is increased causing dilatation of the left atrium and stretching of the patent foramen ovale with more left-to-right shunting at the atrial level, thus, worsening congestive heart failure.

Large patent ductus arteriosus could cause pulmonary vascular obstructive disease, but is not usually treated until after two years of age.

Patients with large shunts are at risk for congestive failure, while those with smaller shunts are at risk for endocarditis, aneurysm, calcification, and paradoxical emboli.

▌ Diagnosis

▌ **Clinical pattern:** patients with small patent ductus arteriosus are asymptomatic; in the presence of patent ductus arteriosus of moderate size, recurrent pulmonary infections can be the only symptom; infants with large patent ductus arteriosus present with congestive heart failure secondary to increase pulmonary blood flow, including easy fatigability (poor feeding), shortness of breath, pallor sweating and cool extremities; signs include bounding pulses, increased left ventricular apical impulse, thrill, continuous murmur and pulmonary sounds consistent with pulmonary edema such as rales and wheezing; the patent ductus arteriosus murmur is best heard over the second left intercostal space; a continuous systolic and diastolic murmur, characterized with a crescendo and decrescendo pattern, peaking at around the closure of the aortic valve (A_2), and clicking noises during the murmur that give the characteristic machinery quality of the patent ductus arteriosus murmur; murmurs mimicking patent ductus arteriosus include AP window, venous hum, ruptured sinus of Valsalva (with aorta to right atrium, right ventricle or left atrium shunts), coronary artery to ventricular cavity fistula and tetralogy of Fallot with pulmonary atresia and large collaterals.

▌ **Electrocardiogram:** in large patent ductus arteriosus left ventricular hypertrophy; if the pulmonary artery pressure is elevated, biventricular hypertrophy.

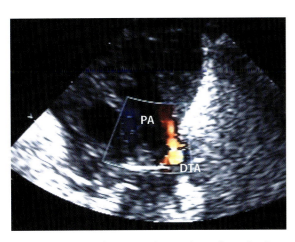

Fig. 1.12.2. Patent ductus arteriosus: echocardiography. Parasternal short axis view in a neonate showing the left-to-right shunt through the patent ductus arteriosus (*DTA* descending thoracic aorta, *PA* pulmonary artery) (photograph courtesy of Dr. Nicole Sekarski)

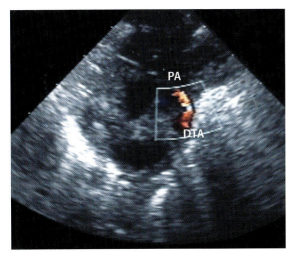

Fig. 1.12.3. Patent ductus arteriosus: echocardiography. Suprasternal short axis view in a neonate showing the left-to-right shunt through the patent ductus arteriosus (*DTA* descending thoracic aorta, *PA* pulmonary artery) (photograph courtesy of Dr. Nicole Sekarski)

■ **Chest X-ray:** enlarged aorta and left atrium as well as left ventricle; in patients with large patent ductus arteriosus there is also dilatation of the pulmonary arteries.

■ **Echocardiogram:** the ductus arteriosus can be seen in the parasternal short axis (Fig. 1.12.2) and the suprasternal (Fig. 1.12.3) views; color flow Doppler shows blood flow across the

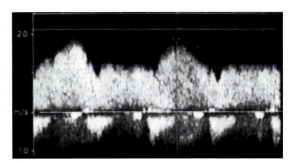

Fig. 1.12.4. Patent ductus arteriosus: echocardiography. Parasternal short axis view in a neonate showing the Doppler flow velocity with continuous left-to-right shunt through the patent ductus arteriosus (photograph courtesy of Dr. Nicole Sekarski)

ductus; the pulmonary arterial pressure can be compared to systemic arterial pressure by assessing the pressure gradient across the ductus using Doppler flow velocity (Fig. 1.12.4).

■ **Cardiac catheterization:** almost never performed in children with isolated patent ductus arteriosus for diagnostic purposes; used in interventional cardiology for coil or device closure; useful in adults to evaluate pulmonary vascular resistance and reactivity.

■ Indications for surgical treatment

The treatment of choice for patent ductus arteriosus after infancy is interventional cardiology with coil or device occlusion whenever possible.

Premature neonates with a patent ductus arteriosus are given a trial of indomethacin, unless renal insufficiency precludes it. Indomethacin treatment is usually given within the first 48 hours of age at a dose of 0.2 mg/kg as a first dose and repeated a second and third time every 12 hours if the ductus arteriosus is still open. In premature babies, a smaller dose of 0.1 mg/kg is given in case of poor renal maturity at that age.

Complications of indomethacin therapy include renal failure, abnormal platelet count and function. Eighty percent of patent ductus arteriosus in premature babies close with indomethacin therapy.

Recently ibuprofen has been successfully introduced for closure of patent ductus arteriosus in premature neonates, particularly in the presence of severe pulmonary hypertension.

Patent ductus arteriosus in premature infants, in whom indomethacin or ibuprofen therapy failed, is not amenable to coil occlusion because of their small size. Surgical closure is indicated in neonates with congestive heart failure and/or dependency on positive pressure ventilation, or those failing to thrive if the ductus remains patent despite indomethacin therapy. Infants in congestive heart failure should be stabilized with medical treatment and then undergo surgical closure.

In children, large ductus arteriosus difficult to close using coils or device requires surgical closure. It is extremely unlikely that a patent ductus arteriosus, even of small size, will spontaneously close after one year of age, and closure should, thus, be recommended.

▌ Surgical treatment

The surgical procedure is performed through a left postero-lateral thoracotomy without cardiopulmonary bypass; occasionally, in adults with large hypertensive patent ductus arteriosus with calcification on the ductal wall, cardiopulmonary bypass may be utilized.

In the case of repair of associated lesions with cardiopulmonary bypass from median sternotomy, the repair of patent ductus arteriosus is performed through a transmediastinal approach; in this case the ductus is exposed by dissecting along the superior aspect of the pulmonary artery bifurcation and closed at the beginning of cardiopulmonary bypass.

After careful dissection from the adjacent tissues, closure of the patent ductus can be obtained by means of ligature (Fig. 1.12.5) or surgical division between two vascular clamps and anastomosis of the two ductal stumps.

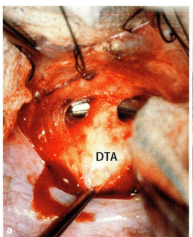
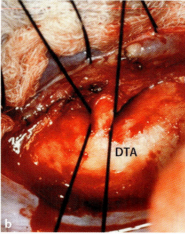
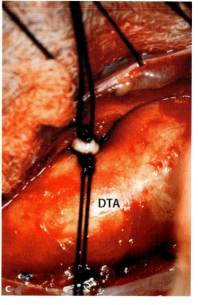

Fig. 1.12.5. Patent ductus arteriosus: surgery. **a** through a postero-lateral left thoracotomy: after division of the hemiazygos vein and longitudinal incision of the mediastinal pleura, the patent ductus arteriosus is dissected free and encircled with a surgical instrument (*DTA* descending thoracic aorta), **b** the patent ductus arteriosus is controlled with two silk ties, **c** the patent ductus arteriosus is doubly ligated with the silk ties

In premature neonates, due to the extreme friability of the ductal tissue, extensive dissection in the area of the patent ductus is avoided, and closure is accomplished with a metal clip.

▮ Potential complications

Residual or recurrent patency (after ligature, not after division), hemorrhage, paradoxical arterial hypertension (in neonates), chylothorax, recurrent nerve lesion.

▮ References

Blalock A (1946) Operative closure of the patent ductus arteriosus. Surg Gynecol Obstet 82:113

Brandt B, Marvin WJ, Ehrenhaft JL, Heintz S, Doty DB (1981) Ligation of patent ductus arteriosus in premature infants. Ann Thorac Surg 32:167

Campbell M (1968) Natural history of patent ductus arteriosus. Br Heart J 30:4

Dooley KJ (1984) Management of the premature infant with a patent ductus arteriosus. Pediatr Clin North Am 31:1159–1174

Fan LL, Campbell DN, Clarke DR, Washington RL, Fix EJ, White CW (1989) Paralyzed left vocal cord associated with ligation of patent ductus arteriosus. J Thorac Cardiovasc Surg 98:611

Fleming WH, Sarafian LB, Kugler JD, Nelson RM (1983) Ligation of patent ductus arteriosus in premature infants: importance of accurate anatomic definition. Pediatrics 71:373–375

Friedman WF, Hirschlau MJ, Printz MP, Pitlick PT, Kirkpatrick SE (1976) Pharmacologic closure of patent ductus arteriosus in the premature infant. N Engl J Med 295:526

Gross RE, Hubbard JP (1939) Surgical ligation of a patent ductus arteriosus. JAMA 112:729–731

Hoffman JIE, Kaplan S (2002) The incidence of congenital heart disease. J Am Coll Cardiol 39:1890–1900

Kron IL, Mentzer RM, Rheuban KS, Nolan SP (1984) A simple, rapid technique for operative closure of patent ductus arteriosus in the premature infant. Ann Thorac Surg 37:422

Marino B, Corno AF, Carotti A, Pasquini L, Giannico S, Guccione P, Bevilacqua M, De Simone G, Marcelletti C (1990) Pediatric cardiac surgery guided by echocardiography. Scand J Thorac Cardiovasc Surg 24:197–201

Nezafati MH, Mahmoodi E, Hashemian SH, Hamedanchi A (2002) Video-assisted thoracoscopic surgical (VATS) closure of patent ductus arteriosus: report of three-hundred cases. Heart Surg Forum 5:57–59

Pham JT, Carlos MA (2002) Current treatment strategies of symptomatic patent ductus arteriosus. J Pediatr Health Care 16:306–310

Pontius RG, Danielson GK, Noonan JA, Judson JP (1981) Illusion leading to surgical closure of the distal left pulmonary artery instead of the ductus arteriosus. J Thorac Cardiovasc Surg 82:107–113

Quinn D, Cooper B, Clyman RI (2002) Factors associated with permanent closure of the ductus arteriosus: a role for prolonged indomethacin therapy. Pediatrics 110:10

Schmidt B, Wright LL, Davis P, Solimano A, Roberts RS (2002) Ibuprofen prophylaxis in preterm neonates. Lancet 360:492

Tokuda Y, Matsumoto M, Sugita T (2001) Optimal treatment for adult patient ductus arteriosis. Ann Thorac Surg 72:2186

Left ventricular outflow tract obstruction

Valvular

■ **Incidence**

Aortic stenosis is rare in infancy. It is present in 0.004–0.34% of live births; 75% of patients are males. It ranks 9th among critical congenital heart diseases in infants (2.9%). Incidence increases with age to become the second most common congenital heart disease after ventricular septal defect in the third decade of life.

■ **Morphology**

The commissures may be fused, the valve ring is occasionally hypoplastic. The orifice of the aortic valve could be eccentric. The valve is commonly bicuspid in aortic stenosis and the leaflets are asymmetric in 40% of cases. Fusion between the right coronary and left coronary cusps will result in a right-to-left commissure, and fusion of right coronary and non-coronary cusps results in antero-posterior commissure. A fusion of the left coronary and non-coronary cusps is extremely rare.

There is occasionally more than one level of obstruction in the left ventricular outflow tract together with aortic valvular stenosis. About 10% of patients with aortic valvular stenosis have subvalvar aortic stenosis. Supravalvar aortic stenosis is rarely associated with aortic stenosis.

In 50% of valvular aortic stenosis cases, there is a certain degree of aortic insufficiency associated with it.

Aortic valvular stenosis is not always the result of a bicuspid aortic valve, since a bicuspid aortic valve is 10–20 times as common as aortic stenosis. Therefore, in a small number of cases, a bicuspid valve will lead to aortic stenosis with the majority not developing into aortic stenosis. Right-to-left commissures have a poorer prognosis in bicuspid aortic valve compared to anteroposterior commissures in developing aortic stenosis. Also eccentric orifices have a poorer prognosis than central orifices in developing aortic stenosis.

■ **Associated anomalies**

Subvalvular and/or supravalvular obstruction, hypoplastic aortic annulus, hypoplastic aortic arch, aortic coarctation, mitral stenosis, mitral regurgitation, atrial septal defect, ventricular septal defect, patent ductus arteriosus. In neonates, relatively frequent association of left ventricular hypoplasia or fibroelastosis.

■ **Pathophysiology**

The left ventricle becomes hypertrophied because of the pressure overload. In severe cases contractility will diminish resulting in heart failure, affecting the left atrial pressure causing pulmonary edema and right heart failure.

The ascending aorta may become dilated due to the forceful jet of blood as it cross the aortic valve.

If significant aortic regurgitation is associated with stenosis, left ventricular failure and dilation will develop faster.

∎ **Natural history:** Mild cases usually do not progress. Moderate and severe cases usually do progress. Sudden death may occur to any patient with aortic stenosis but mainly to symptomatic patients.

∎ Diagnosis

∎ **Clinical pattern:** when the children are asymptomatic, the murmur detected is typically at a routine physical examination; in the minority of patients there is complaint of chest pain which is angina-like, with syncope particularly during exercise; physical examination is benign except for a palpable thrill particularly over the suprasternal notch as well as the right second intercostal space; on auscultation the first heart sound is normal; there is an ejection click followed by a harsh systolic crescendo-decrescendo type murmur; the second heart sound is normal except with severe aortic stenosis where the aortic valve closure (A_2) will be delayed secondary to prolonged left ventricular systole causing reversed splitting or single S_2; symptomatic neonates with severe stenosis present with tachypnea and congestive heart failure; progressive metabolic acidosis; some neonates with critical aortic stenosis present in a state of cardiovascular collapse, with severe hepatomegaly, impalpable peripheral pulses and progressive metabolic acidosis.

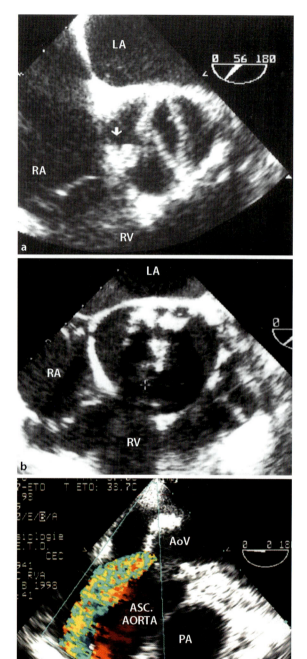

Fig. 1.13.1. Aortic valve stenosis: echocardiography. **a** transesophageal view showing a transversal section of the aortic valve, with fusion of two leaflets with the largest one having a thick median raphe (*LA* left atrium, *RA* right atrium, *RV* right ventricle, white arrow=median raphe), **b** transesophageal view showing a transversal section of a bicuspid aortic valve with thick leaflets and complete fusion of one commissura, **c** transesophageal color Doppler with a stenotic bicuspid aortic valve doming in systole towards the ascending aorta (*ASC. AORTA* ascending aorta, *AoV* aortic valve, *PA* pulmonary artery) (photographs courtesy of Dr. Pierre-Guy Chassot)

▌ **Electrocardiogram:** left ventricular hypertrophy with possibly ST and T wave changes, particularly in the inferolateral leads; the changes on the electrocardiogram reflects the daily strain (i.e., chronic) of the myocardium rather than the severity at rest.

▌ **Chest X-ray:** mild cardiomegaly with a prominent aortic arch.

▌ **Echocardiogram:** generally diagnostic (Fig. 1.13.1), the short axis reveals the aortic valve ring and the left ventricular outflow tract which should be assessed; pulsed and continuous Doppler allows estimation of transvalvular pressure gradients; in addition, the presence and degree of aortic insufficiency should be evaluated, and this is best seen with color Doppler or Doppler flow in the apical four chamber and parasternal long axis views; the severity of aortic insufficiency is assessed by the width of the aortic insufficiency jet and flow in the descending aorta (diminished and severe aortic insufficiency with reversal flow in diastole).

▌ **Cardiac catheterization:** cardiac catheterization is performed when:
▌ percutaneous balloon valvuloplasty is intended,
▌ with angina, ST-T changes in stress or rest ECG, to evaluate left ventricular pressures and coronary blood flow,
▌ fainting spells, to evaluate the left ventricular outflow tract,
▌ to quantitate the left ventricular volume.

Left and right anterior oblique views are good to visualize the aortic valve and the left ventricular outflow tract.

▌ Indications for surgical treatment

In infants with critical aortic stenosis the aim is to improve cardiac output.

In older children the aim is to preserve the myocardium against irreversible damage.

The following criteria are used to decide intervention:
▌ Transvalvular pressure gradient
▌ Episode of syncope
▌ Angina
▌ Premature ventricular contractions
▌ ST and T changes
▌ Echocardiographic evidence of left ventricular dysfunction.

More than 50 mmHg pressure gradient with no aortic insufficiency may benefit from balloon valvuloplasty. Balloon valvuloplasty and surgical valvotomy results are comparable.

Aortic valve replacement with a prosthetic valve is indicated with aortic stenosis and aortic insufficiency when the aortic insufficiency appears to be problematic as much as aortic stenosis. Aortic valve replacement is also indicated in severely deformed aortic valves. Children might benefit from the Ross operation.

In the presence of aortic valvular stenosis with hypoplastic aortic annulus, aortic valve replacement with enlargement of the aortic annulus is required.

▌ Surgical treatment (on cardiopulmonary bypass)

After a transversal or an oblique aortotomy, the aortic valvotomy is performed accordingly with the aortic valve morphology: the fused commissures are opened by a careful incision not reaching the aortic wall (Fig. 1.13.2). The obtained opening is controlled with Hegar dilators and compared with the normal size for the age and body weight.

Aortic valve replacement, where required, can be performed with conventional surgical technique or even better with a Ross operation (Fig. 1.13.3) (autotransplantation of the native pulmonary valve in aortic position and right ventricle to pulmonary artery continuity obtained with valved homograft or heterograft) if the size of the aortic annulus is adequate, or it may require enlargement of the aortic annulus with one of the following techniques:

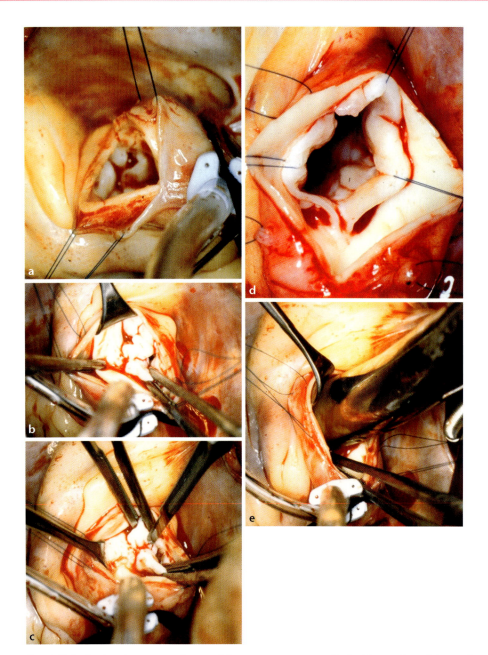

Fig. 1.13.2. Aortic valvotomy. **a** after an oblique aortotomy, exposure of the aortic valve, **b** exposure of the fused commissures of the tri-leaflet aortic valve, **c** the fused commissures are opened by a careful incision not reaching the aortic wall, **d** wide opening of the aortic valve after incision of the commissures, **e** the obtained opening is controlled with Hegar dilators and compared with the normal size for the age and body weight

▮ Posterior annular enlargement
- Nicks: aortotomy extended through the non-coronary sinus and the anterior leaflet of the mitral valve; enlargement obtained with prosthetic patch.
- Managouian: aortotomy extended through the left and non-coronary si-

nuses and the anterior leaflet of the mitral valve; enlargement obtained with prosthetic patch.
▮ Aorto-ventriculoplasty
- Konno-Rastan (Fig. 1.13.4): aortotomy extended through the right ventricular outflow tract, aortic annulus divided

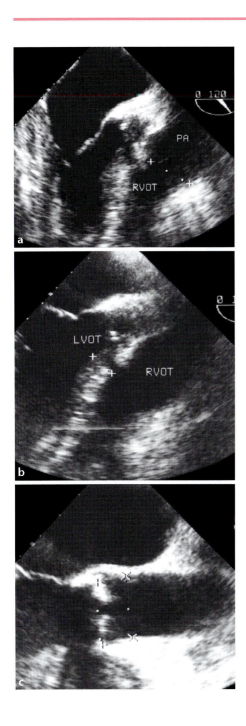

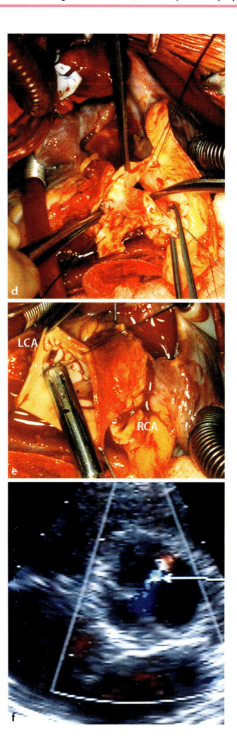

Fig. 1.13.3. Ross operation: intra-operative evaluation. **a** transesophageal echocardiography showing the measurement of the diameter of the pulmonary valve annulus (*PA* pulmonary artery, *RVOT* right ventricular outflow tract), **b** transesophageal echocardiography showing the measurement of the thickness of the interventricular septum (*LVOT* left ventricular outflow tract, *RVOT* right ventricular outflow tract), **c** transesophageal echocardiography showing the measurement of the diameter of the aortic valve at the level of the annulus and of the sinotubular junction, **d** resection of the native stenotic aortic valve, after previous balloon dilatation, **e** implantation of the pulmonary autograft, with reimplantation of the left coronary artery; the right coronary artery, already prepared, is ready to be reimplanted (*LCA* left coronary artery, *RCA* right coronary artery), **f** transesophageal echocardiography showing a trivial leakage (white arrow) through the pulmonary autograft implanted in the aortic position (photographs courtesy of Dr. Pierre-Guy Chassot)

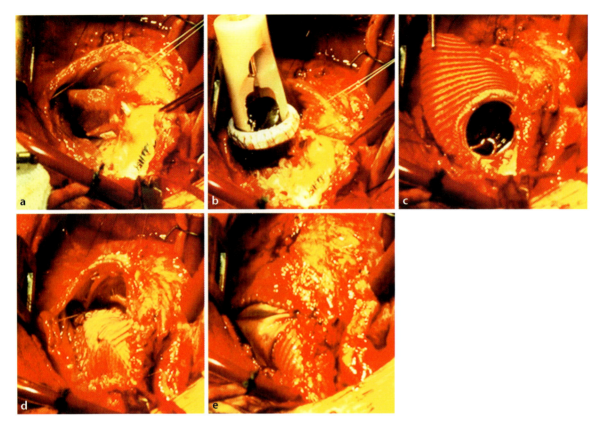

Fig. 1.13.4. Konno-Rastan operation. **a** aortotomy extended through the right ventricular outflow tract, division of the aortic annulus between the right and left cusps, incision of the interventricular septum, **b** insertion of a mechanical valve on the native aortic annulus, **c** the insertion of the mechanical valve on the new aortic annulus is completed with more than half of the valve circumference inserted on the Dacron patch enlarging the interventricular septum and the aortic annulus, **d** the Dacron patch used to enlarge the interventricular septum and the aortic annulus is used to enlarge the aortic root, **e** the operation is completed with the anastomosis of the pericardial patch to enlarge the incised right ventricular outflow tract

between right and left cusps, interventricular septum incised; enlargement obtained with two patches, one to enlarge interventricular septum, aortic annulus and aortic root, the second one to enlarge the incised right ventricular outflow tract.

– Clarke: aorto-ventriculoplasty performed using an aortic homograft instead of an artificial valve; the septal leaflet of the mitral valve of the homograft is used as a patch for the incised interventricular septum.

– Ross-Konno: aorto-ventriculoplasty performed using a pulmonary autograft.

∎ Potential complications

Residual or recurrent aortic valve stenosis, aortic valve regurgitation, complete atrioventricular block.

∎ Sub-valvular

∎ Incidence

Isolated subaortic stenosis comprises 0.5% of all congenital heart diseases.

■ Morphology

The subaortic obstruction can be determined by the following different morphological types:

■ Posterior malalignment of the outlet septum;

■ Asymmetric septal hypertrophy, or hypertrophic cardiomyopathy;

■ Discrete fibromuscular diaphragm or ridge, generally close to the aortic valve;

■ Extensive fibro-muscular tunnel, with involvement of the mitral valve;

■ Any combination of the above.

The aortic annulus can be normal or hypoplastic.

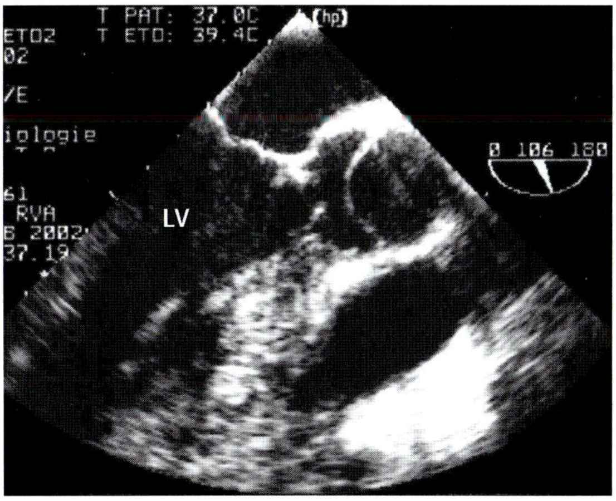

Fig. 1.13.5. Sub-valvular aortic stenosis: echocardiography. Transesophageal view showing the left ventricular outflow tract with a fibromuscular diaphragm close to the aortic valve (*LV* left ventricle) (photograph courtesy of Dr. Pierre-Guy Chassot)

■ Associated anomalies

Coarctation of the aorta, aortic arch interruption, mitral stenosis, ventricular septal defect, atrioventricular septal defect, double chamber right ventricle, univentricular heart.

■ Pathophysiology

The pathophysiologic pattern is similar to the valvular stenosis, with the difference that in subvalvular obstruction the aortic valve leaflets may be damaged by the stenosis jet, causing deformity of the aortic valve and aortic regurgitation.

The aortic valve regurgitation seems to be progressive, in the absence of surgical treatment of the subaortic obstruction, particularly in the presence of the discrete fibromuscular diaphragm.

■ Diagnosis

■ **Clinical pattern:** usually asymptomatic; congestive heart failure as seen in severe valvar aortic stenosis is not common here; systolic murmur heard over the base of the heart or left upper sternal border with or without diastolic aortic regurgitation murmur; aortic regurgitation is not severe when present.

■ **Electrocardiogram:** left ventricular hypertrophy; changes are not as prominent as with valvar aortic valvular stenosis.

■ **Chest X-ray:** cardiomegaly is sometimes noted, but not as severe as with valvular stenosis.

■ **Echocardiogram:** this shows the type and extent of the left ventricular outflow tract obstruction and can assess the pressure gradient and presence and the degree of aortic regurgitation (Fig. 1.13.5); aortic valve is noted to close early in systole which is most probably secondary to turbulent flow in the left ventricular outflow tract.

■ **Cardiac catheterization:** performed in order to rule out or quantify associated lesions.

■ Indications for surgical treatment

Surgery is eventually indicated in all cases. Resection of the discrete fibromuscular diaphragm or wedge of muscle from the fibromuscular tunnel when the pressure gradient is more than 30 mmHg, or at the first appearance of aortic valve regurgitation not seen previously. In the presence of an extensive fibro-muscular tunnel, the surgical treatment depends on the presence of a normal or small aortic annulus. Left ventricle to aorta valved conduit has been practically abandoned because of its disappointing results.

■ Surgical treatment (on cardiopulmonary bypass)

The discrete fibromuscular diaphragm is treated by diaphragm dissection/resection (Fig. 1.13.6) with septal myotomy/myectomy; in the presence of malalignment between the left ventricular outflow tract and the ascending aorta, septal myectomy is needed in order to obtain a straight outflow and prevent recurrencies.

Extensive fibro-muscular tunnel is treated with two different techniques, depending on the size of the aortic annulus:

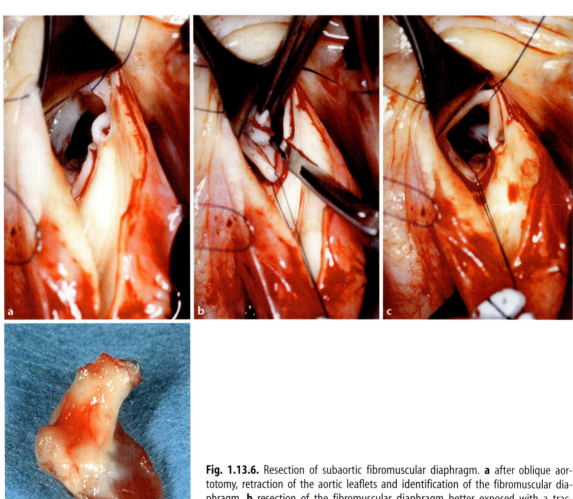

Fig. 1.13.6. Resection of subaortic fibromuscular diaphragm. **a** after oblique aortotomy, retraction of the aortic leaflets and identification of the fibromuscular diaphragm, **b** resection of the fibromuscular diaphragm better exposed with a traction suture, **c** after resection of the fibromuscular diaphragm and myectomy, inspection of the subaortic area and the anterior leaflet of the mitral valve, with retraction of the aortic leaflets, **d** result of resection of the fibromuscular diaphragm and myectomy

▮ Small annulus: aorto-ventriculoplasty (see above for aortic valve replacement).

▮ Normal annulus: ventricular septoplasty, generally called partial Konno-Rastan procedure, even if described the first time by Cooley in 1986; the right ventricular outflow tract and the interventricular septum are incised, without incising the aortic annulus; relief of subaortic obstruction is obtained with a prosthetic patch to enlarge the interventricular septum; a second patch is required to enlarge the incised right ventricular outflow tract.

▮ Potential complications

Residual or recurrent left ventricular outflow tract obstruction, residual or recurrent aortic valve regurgitation, mitral valve lesion, creation of ventricular septal defect, complete atrioventricular block.

Supra-valvular

▮ Incidence

This very rare congenital heart defect, the less frequent type of aortic stenosis, is common in patients with Williams-Beuren syndrome: elfin facies, mental retardation, dental problems, infantile hypercalcemia.

▮ Morphology

Supra-valvular aortic stenosis may be localized or diffuse:

▮ *Localized*: usually there is an externally apparent waisting of the supra-valvular area of aorta, just above or at the upper level of attachments of the valve leaflets; in association with some dilatation of the sinuses of Valsalva, there is an hourglass appearance. There is a variable amount of intimal thickening, with an internal shelf which substantially increases the obstruc-

tion and may cause a severe stenosis or even a complete occlusion of the origin of the left main coronary artery.

▮ *Diffuse*: less frequently the supra-valvular narrowing is diffuse, with extension through the entire ascending aorta, even beyond into the aortic arch and the origin of the brachiocephalic arteries.

▮ Associated anomalies

One-third of all cases have Williams-Beuren syndrome. Thickened aortic valve leaflets but without a true valvular stenosis (30%), rarely hypoplastic aortic annulus or subvalvular obstruction, hypoplastic pulmonary arteries (30%), coarctation of the aorta (15%), stenosis at the origin of the subclavian and carotid arteries or renal artery stenosis (5%), very rarely ventricular septal defect.

Obstruction of the origin of the left main coronary artery is more frequent, but it can also occur in the right main coronary artery. In the absence of obstruction at the origin, the coronary arteries are exposed to high pressure and as a consequence they present with dilatations, tortuosities and medial hypertrophy.

▮ Pathophysiology

The only difference with the valvular aortic stenosis consists in the fact that the coronary arteries are exposed to high pressure due to the localization of the obstruction distally to the origin of the coronary arteries.

▮ Diagnosis

▮ **Clinical pattern:** symptoms rarely develop in infancy, more frequently in childhood; they are similar to the valvular aortic stenosis, although angina pectoris may be more frequent because of the increased incidence

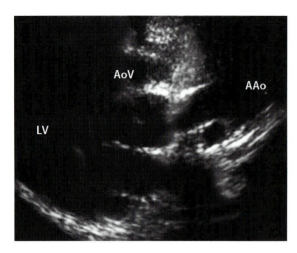

Fig. 1.13.7. Supra-valvular aortic stenosis: echocardiography. Long axis view showing the left ventricular outflow tract with normal aortic valve and narrowing of the supra-valvular area of aorta, just above the attachments of the valve leaflets, in association with some dilatation of the sinuses of Valsalva (*AAo* ascending aorta, *AoV* aortic valve, *LV* left ventricle) (photograph courtesy of Dr. Nicole Sekarski)

of early onset of coronary atherosclerosis; auscultation: the main difference with valvular stenosis is that the systolic murmur is sited higher; the blood pressure is higher in the left arm than in the right arm (koanda effect).

▮ **Electrocardiogram:** similar to the valvular stenosis.

▮ **Chest X-ray:** similar to the valvular stenosis.

▮ **Echocardiogram:** diagnosis of supra-valvular stenosis and identification of the type and degree of obstruction can be obtained with echocardiography (Fig. 1.13.7).

▮ **Cardiac catheterization:** cardiac catheterization is indicated in order to:
- localize the site of pressure drop by withdrawing the catheter from the aorta to the left ventricle
- show the morphology by angiography
- identify associated anomalies.

▮ Indications for surgical treatment

Progression of the supra-valvular aortic stenosis has been documented, more rapid and severe than in valvular stenosis.

Operation is indicated in the presence of pressure gradient of 50 mmHg or more, at whatever age, in view of the progressive nature of the lesion.

▮ Surgical treatment (on cardiopulmonary bypass)

▮ *Localized type*:
- classical technique: the aorta is opened above the valve and the incision is prolonged into the right coronary sinus, into the non-coronary sinus or into both the right and non-coronary sinuses. After inspection of the origin of the coronary arteries, the intimal shelf is resected. Aortic enlargement is then obtained with either a diamond-shaped (in the case of a single incision in one of the sinuses of Valsalva) or with an inverted-Y (in the case of incision extended into both the right and non-coronary sinuses) prosthetic patch.
- Brom technique: the aorta is completely transected just above the supra-valvular stenosis. All three sinuses of Valsalva are then incised and enlarged with three separate prosthetic patches. The ascending aorta is then reconstructed with end-to-end anastomosis.

▮ *Diffuse type*:
Deep hypothermia and circulatory arrest are generally required. The incision in correspondence of the supra-valvular obstruction is prolonged through the entire ascending aorta and aortic arch, rarely until the descending thoracic aorta, to find a normal diameter of the aorta. Enlargement is obtained with a prosthetic patch or with an aortic homograft.

■ Potential complications

Residual or recurrent supra-valvular stenosis, aortic valve regurgitation, coronary artery lesion.

■ References

Alexiou C, McDonald A, Langley SM, Dalrymple-Hay MJ, Haw MP, Monro JL (2000) Aortic valve replacement in children: are mechanical prostheses a good option? Eur J Cardiothorac Surg 17:125–133

Bacha EA, Satou GM, Moran AM, Zurakowski D, Marx GR, Keane JF, Jonas RA (2001) Valve-spearing operation for balloon-induced aortic regurgitation in congenital aortic stenosis. J Thorac Cardiovasc Surg 122:162–168

Beuren AJ, Apitz J, Harmjanz D (1962) Supravalvular aortic stenosis in association with mental retardation and certain facial appearance. Circulation 26:1235–1240

Calhoon JH, Bolton JW (1995) Ross/Konno procedure for critical aortic stenosis in infancy. Ann Thorac Surg 60:597–599

Campbell M (1968) The natural history of congenital aortic stenosis. Br Heart J 30:514

Cicini MP, Giannico S, Iorio FS, Giamberti A, Corno AF, Marino B, Marcelletti C (1990) Stenosi sottoaortica post-chirurgica dopo chiusura di difetto interventricolare. G Ital Cardiol 20(Suppl II):43

Cicini MP, Giannico S, Marino B, Iorio FS, Corno AF, Marcelletti C (1992) Acquired subvalvular aortic stenosis after repair of a ventricular septal defect. Chest 101:115–118

Clarke DR (1987) Extended aortic root replacement for treatment of left ventricular outflow tract obstruction. J Cardiac Surg 2(Suppl):121

Cooley DA, Norman JC, Reul GJ, Kidd JN, Nihill MR (1976) Surgical treatment of left ventricular outflow tract obstruction with apico-aortic valved conduit. Surgery 80:674

Cooley DA, Garrett JR (1986) Septoplasty for left ventricular outflow obstruction without aortic valve replacement: a new technique. Ann Thorac Surg 42:445

Corno AF, Marcelletti C, Losekoot TG, Becker AE (1980) Aortoventricoloplastica e condotti valvolati: techniche chirurgiche non convenzionali per ostruzioni all'efflusso ventricolare sinistro estese. Arch Chir Torac Cardiovasc 2:150–151

Corno AF, Giamberti A, Giannico S, Marino B, Picardo S, Ballerini L, Marcelletti C (1988) Long-term results after extracardiac valved conduits implanted for complex congenital heart disease. J Card Surg 3:495–500

Corno AF, George B, Williams RG, Laks H (1990) Valve re-replacement in children. J Am Coll Cardiol 15:179A

Corno AF, Zoia E, Santoro F, Camesasca C, Biagioli B, Grossi A (1992) Epicardial damage induced by topical cooling during pediatric cardiac surgery. Br Heart J 67:174–176

Corno AF, von Segesser LK (1999) Is hypothermia necessary in pediatric cardiac surgery? Eur J Cardiothorac Surg 15:110–111

Corno AF, Goy JJ, Hurni M, Sekarski N, Payot M, von Segesser LK (2000) Evolving concept of treatment for aortic valve stenosis. Thorac Cardiovasc Surg 48(Suppl I):93

Corno AF (2000) Surgery for congenital heart disease. Curr Opinion Cardiol 15:238–243

Corno AF, Goy JJ, Hurni M, Payot M, Sekarski N, von Segesser LK (2001) Treatment of congenital aortic valve stenosis: impact of the Ross operation. Swiss Med Wkly 131:65–69

Corno AF, Hurni M, Griffin H, Jeanrenaud X, von Segesser LK (2001) Glutaraldehyde-fixed bovine jugular vein as a substitute for the pulmonary valve in the Ross operation. J Thorac Cardiovasc Surg 122:493–494

Corno AF, Chassot PG, Jeanrenaud X, Tozzi P, Wicky S, von Segesser LK (2002) Aortic valve disease: is the Ross operation the solution? Med Cardiovasc 5(Suppl):4–46

Corno AF, Chassot PG, Hurni M, Jeanrenaud X, Tozzi P, von Segesser LK (2002) Ross operation: consistent medium-term results. Cardiovasc Engin 1:91

Corno AF, von Segesser LK (2003) The stealth Ross operation. Asian Cardiovasc Thorac Ann (in press)

Davtyan HG, Corno AF, Drinkwater DC, George B, Laks H (1986) Valve replacement for congenital heart disease. Circulation 74:II-250

Detter C, Fischlein T, Feldmeier C, Nollert G, Reichart B (2001) Aortic valvotomy for congenital valvular aortic stenosis: a 37-year experience. Ann Thorac Surg 71:1564–1571

Doty DB, Polansky DB, Jenson CB (1977) Supravalvular aortic stenosis. Repair by extended aortoplasty. J Thorac Cardiovasc Surg 74:362

Edwards JE (1965) Pathology of left ventricular outflow tract obstruction. Circulation 31:586–599

Elkins RC, Knott-Craig CJ, Ward KE, Lane MM (1998) The Ross operation in children: 10-year experience. Ann Thorac Surg 65:496–502

Erez E, Kanter KR, Tam VK, Williams WH (2002) Konno aortoventriculoplasty in children and adolescents: from prosthetic valves to the Ross operation. Ann Thorac Surg 74:122–126

Freedom RM, Fowler RS, Duncan WJ (1981) Rapid evolution from normal left ventricular outflow tract to fatal subaortic stenosis in infancy. Br Heart J 45:605–609

Freedom RM (1989) Balloon therapy of critical aortic stenosis in the neonate. The therapeutic conundrum resolved? Circulation 80:1087–1088

Fyler DC, Buckley LP, Hellenbrand WE, Cohn HE (1980) Report of the New England Regional Infant Care Program. Pediatrics 65(Suppl):375–461

Gatzoulis MA, Rigby ML, Shinebourne EA, Redington AN (1995) Contemporary results of balloon valvuloplasty and surgical valvotomy for congenital aortic stenosis. Arch Dis Child 73:66–69

Hoffman JIE, Kaplan S (2002) The incidence of congenital heart disease. J Am Coll Cardiol 39:1890–1900

Horisberger J, Jegger D, Boone Y, Seigneul I, Pierrel N, Hurni M, Corno AF, von Segesser LK (1999) Impact of a remote pump head on neonatal priming volumes. Perfusion 14:351–356

Hurni M, Corno AF, Tucker OP, Payot M, Sekarski N, Cotting J, Bernath MA, von Segesser LK (2000) Venpro: a new pulmonary valved conduit. Thorac Cardiovasc Surg 48(Suppl I):120

Khanna SK, Anstadt MP, Bhimji S, Bannan MM, Mawulawde K, Zumbro GL, Moore HV (2002) Apico-aortic conduits in children with severe left ventricular outflow tract obstruction. Ann Thorac Surg 73:81–86

Konno S, Imai Y, Iida Y, Nakajima M, Tatsuno K (1975) A new method for prosthetic valve replacement in congenital aortic stenosis associated with hypoplasia of the aortic valve ring. J Thorac Cardiovasc Surg 70:909

Lakier JB, Lewis AB, Heymann MA, Stanger P, Hoffman JI, Rudolph AM (1974) Isolated aortic stenosis in the neonate. Natural history and hemodynamic considerations. Circulation 50:801–808

Laudito A, Brook MM, Suleman S, Bleiweis MS, Thompson LD, Hanlye FL, Reddy VM (2001) The Ross procedure in children and young adults: a word of caution. J Thorac Cardiovasc Surg 122:147–153

Marcelletti C, Corno F, Losekoot TG, Olthof H, Schuller J, Bulterijs AHK, Becker AE (1980) Condotti extracardiaci: indicazioni, tecniche e risultati immediati. G Ital Cardiol 10:1041–1054

Marcelletti C, Corno AF (1981) Extracardiac conduits: indications, techniques and early results. 33th Herhalings Cursus Kindergeneeskunde, Amsterdam (Abstracts)

Marino B, De Biase L, Gagliardi MG, Cipriani A, Corno AF, Annichiarico M (1987) Echocardiography in aortic valve disease in the child. In: D'Alessandro LC (ed) Heart Surgery. pp 393–401

Marino B, Corno AF, Carotti A, Pasquini L, Giannico S, Guccione P, Bevilacqua M, De Simone G,

Marcelletti C (1990) Pediatric cardiac surgery guided by echocardiography. Scand J Thorac Cardiovasc Surg 24:197–201

McKay R, Ross DN (1982) Technique for the relief of discrete subaortic stenosis. J Thorac Cardiovasc Surg 84:917

Morrow AG, Fort L, Roberts WL, Braunwald E (1965) Discrete subaortic stenosis complicated by aortic valvular regurgitation. Clinical, hemodynamic, and pathological studies and the results of operative treatment. Circulation 31:163

Ohye RG, Gomet CA, Ohye BJ, Goldberg CS, Bove EL (2001) The Ross/Konno procedure in neonates and infants: intermediate-term survival and autograft function. Ann Thorac Surg 72:823–830

Oswalt JD (1999) Acceptance and versatility of the Ross procedure. Curr Opinion Cardiol 14:90–94

Pierli C, Marino B, Picardo S, Corno AF, Pasquini L, Marcelletti C (1989) Discrete subaortic stenosis: surgery in children based on two dimensional and Doppler echocardiography. Chest 96:325–328

Presbitero P, Somerville J, Revel-Chion R, Ross DN (1982) Open aortic valvotomy for congenital aortic stenosis: late results. Br Heart J 47:26–34

Rastan H, Koncz J (1976) Aortoventriculoplasty. A new technique for the treatment of left ventricular outflow tract obstruction. J Thorac Cardiovasc Surg 71:920

Reddy VM, Rajasinghe HA, Teitel DF, Haas GS, Hanley FL (1996) Aortoventriculoplasty with the pulmonary autograft: the Ross-Konno procedure. J Thorac Cardiovasc Surg 111:158–165

Ross DN (1967) Replacement of aortic and mitral valve with a pulmonary autograft. Lancet 2:956

Santoro F, Corno AF, Papa M, Zoia E (1991) Ostruzioni congenite al tratto di efflusso ventricolare sinistro. G Ital Cardiol 21(Suppl II):39

Shone JD, Sellers RD, Anderson RC, Adams P, Lillehei CW, Edwards JE (1963) The developmental complex of parachute mitral valve, supravalvular ring of left atrium, subaortic stenosis and coarctation of the aorta. Am J Cardiol 11:714–725

Somerville J (1979) Congenital heart disease: changes in form and function. Br Heart J 41:1–22

Somerville J (1985) Fixed subaortic stenosis: a frequently misunderstood lesion. Int J Cardiol 8:145–148

Williams JCP, Barrat-Boyes BG, Lowe JB (1961) Supravalvular aortic stenosis. Circulation 24:1311

Wright GB, Keane JF, Nadas AS, Bernhard WF, Castaneda AR (1983) Fixed subaortic stenosis in the young: medical and surgical course in 83 patients. Am J Cardiol 52:830–835

▮ Incidence

Aortic coarctation, the 7th most common congenital heart defect, is present in 4.6% of all congenital heart diseases, and it is the predominant feature in 0.2–0.6/1000 live births. Aortic coarctation is more frequent in males.

▮ Morphology (Fig. 1.14.1)

Aortic coarctation is a congenital narrowing of the aortic lumen, usually situated between the origin of the left subclavian artery proximally and the junction of the aorta and the ductus arteriosus distally. When the coarctation is an isolated finding, the wall of the aorta is pinched in a waist-like fashion, the ascending and descending portions of the arch tending to expand above and below the site of coarctation. The narrowing may consist of an elongated and diffuse tract, proximally to the ductus arteriosus, or of a sharp constriction in the area of aortic insertion of the arterial duct, with a diaphragmatic shelf of fibrous tissue protruding into the lumen, often with a pin-hole orifice representing the only communication between the ascending and descending aortic segments (Fig. 1.14.2). Aortic arch hypoplasia of mild or severe degree may be present. Collateral circulation between the aorta proximal and distal to the coarctation is increasing in size and extensiveness as the patient ages.

Occasionally the aorta may be redundant and severely kinked opposite the ligamentum arteriosum, without any pressure gradient or with a mild gradient: the so-called pseudocoarctation.

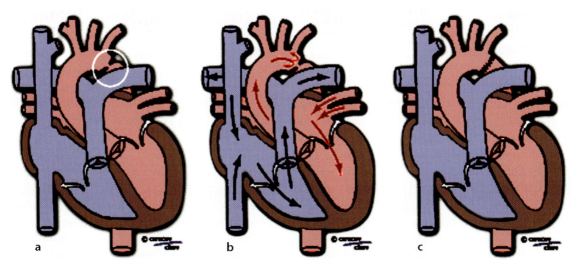

Fig. 1.14.1. Aortic coarctation: **a** morphology, **b** pathophysiology, **c** surgery

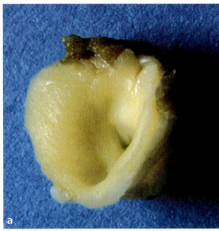

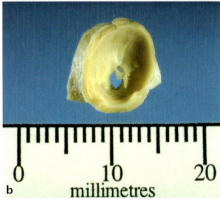

Fig. 1.14.2. Aortic coarctation: morphology. **a** surgically resected aortic isthmus with a pin-hole orifice representing the only communication between the ascending and descending aortic segments, **b** surgically resected aortic isthmus, after an attempt at balloon dilatation: intima lesion corresponding to the orifice represents the only communication between the ascending and descending aortic segments

▮ Associated anomalies

Patent ductus arteriosus, atrial septal defect, atrioventricular septal defect, ventricular septal defect, double inlet ventricle (with or without actual or potential systemic outlet obstruction), supravalvular or valvular mitral stenosis, valvular or subvalvular aortic stenosis (frequently with bicuspid aortic valve), multiple stenotic lesions of the left heart (= Shone's syndrome), transposition of the great arteries (usually with ventricular septal defect, with or without actual or potential systemic outlet obstruction), double-outlet right ventricle (usually with ventricular septal defect, with or without actual or potential systemic outlet obstruction), truncus arteriosus, double discordance, hypoplastic left heart, anomalous origin of coronary arteries, anomalous right subclavian artery, intracranial aneurysms, very rarely tetralogy of Fallot.

▮ Pathophysiology

The position, as related to the ductus arteriosus, determines the pathophysiology, as does patency and closure of the ductus arteriosus, changes in pulmonary vascular resistance, presence of associated lesions, and extent of collateral circulation.

As the narrowing becomes significant more and more collaterals develop. The amount of collaterals may be so large that it will decrease any pressure gradient across the coarctation, and lower extremity blood pressures will be close to the upper extremity blood pressures. The pressure gradient across the coarctation may be more than the difference between the upper and lower extremity blood pressure due to collateral vessels bypassing the area of coarctation.

Neonates (and small infants). In the presence of patent ductus arteriosus, elevated pulmonary resistance maintains systolic right-to-left shunt through the ductus (ductal dependence of the distal systemic circulation, right ventricular pressure overload); the reduction of pulmonary vascular resistance and/or the ductal closure determines poor perfusion of the lower body and particularly inadequate renal perfusion (metabolic acidosis).

Children and adults. Upper body hypertension, with left ventricular pressure overload.

With associated ventricular septal defect. Significant left-to-right intraventricular shunt, with increased pulmonary blood flow and pulmonary hypertension (biventricular pressure and volume overload).

▮ Diagnosis

On examination a murmur is heard over the precordium and back (left interscapular space). The murmur is systolic, but due to the fact that systolic flow at the site of coarctation is slightly after systole ends, i.e., closure of the aortic and pulmonary valves, the murmur appears to spill over into diastole.

▮ Clinical pattern
– neonates: severe congestive heart failure, poor peripheral perfusion, metabolic acidosis, oliguria;
– children: frequently asymptomatic, rarely signs of systemic upper body hypertension, weak or absent femoral pulses;
– adults: endocarditis, aneurysm of intercostal arteries, cerebrovascular accidents, and left ventricle failure.

▮ Electrocardiogram
– neonates: right ventricular hypertrophy, right axis deviation;
– children and adults: normal or left ventricular hypertrophy;
– adults: sometimes ST-T changes.

▮ Chest X-ray
– neonates: cardiomegaly, lung congestion, (rare) pulmonary edema;
– children: normal or mild cardiomegaly, rib notching in older children (and adults).

▮ Echocardiogram
– detection of morphology of the aortic isthmus and of the aortic arch (Fig. 1.14.3); Doppler-derived pressure gradient across the coarctation site; research of associated anomalies; in measuring the pressure gradient across the aortic arch the Doppler flow velocity prior to the point of coarctation should be taken into consideration, especially when calculating the pressure gradient, otherwise the pressure difference would be exaggerated; normally, flow in the descending aorta has a rapid upstroke in systole and brief retro-

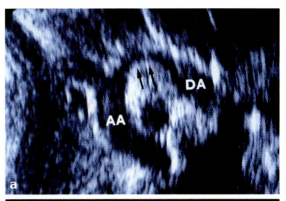
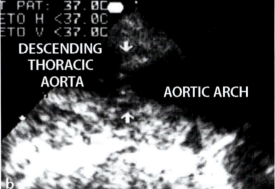
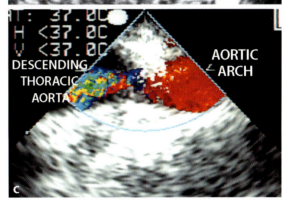

Fig. 1.14.3. Aortic coarctation: echocardiography. **a** suprasternal projection showing the aortic coarctation and the hypoplasia of the aortic arch (black arrows) (*AA* ascending aorta, *DA* descending aorta), **b** transesophageal view showing the fibrous narrowing (white arrows) in correspondence of the aortic isthmus (photograph courtesy of Dr. Pierre-Guy Chassot), **c** transesophageal color Doppler showing the change in flow corresponding to the aortic isthmus (photograph courtesy of Dr. Pierre-Guy Chassot)

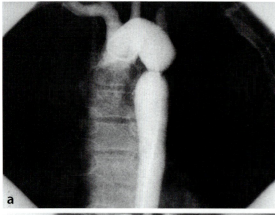

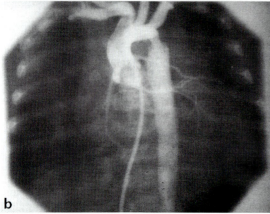

Fig. 1.14.4. Aortic coarctation: angiography. **a** Contrast injection in the ascending aorta showing opacification of the aortic arch, with a sharp constriction in the area of aortic isthmus, **b** contrast injection in the ascending aorta showing opacification of a relatively hypoplastic aortic arch, with a further size reduction in the area of the aortic isthmus

grade flow in early diastole, while in the coarctation the systolic upstroke is reduced with continuous forward flow in diastole.

■ Cardiac catheterization: very limited to

– morphology of the aortic coarctation (Fig. 1.14.4) and of the aortic arch (in case of arch hypoplasia);
– complex associated cardiac lesions, especially if surgical treatment is not confined to coarctectomy.

■ Indications for surgical treatment

Surgery is the treatment of choice and the earlier it is done the better.

■ **Neonates:** emergency surgery, with or without a previous period of medical stabilization (PGE infusion, mechanical ventilation, correction of acidosis).

■ **Infants:** surgery after establishing diagnosis.

■ **Children:** elective surgery.

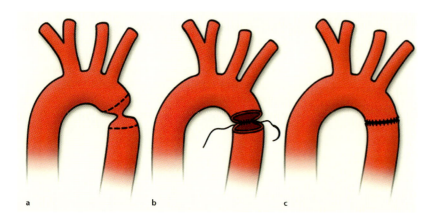

Fig. 1.14.5. Resection and end-to-end anastomosis. **a** incisions proximally and distally to the coarctation to resect the narrowing, **b** anastomosis of the posterior wall, **c** completed anastomosis

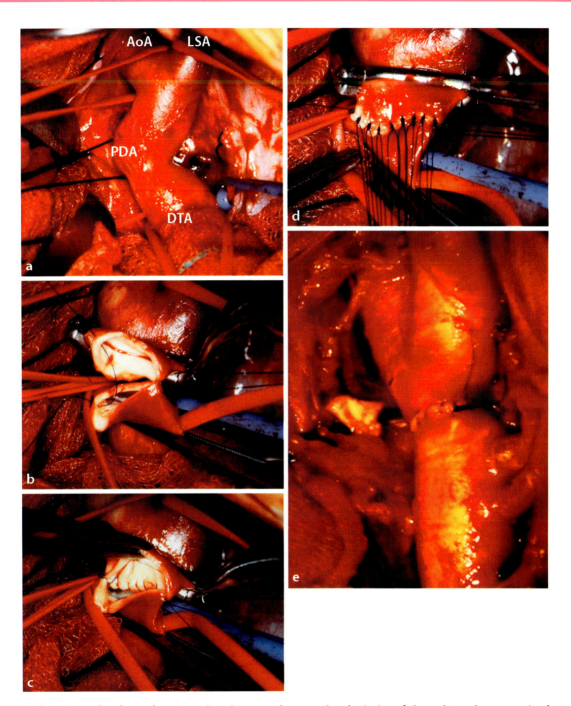

Fig. 1.14.6. Resection and end-to-end anastomosis. **a** intra-operative photograph (postero-lateral left thoracotomy) showing the aortic coarctation. Aortic arch (*AoA*), left subclavian artery (*LSA*) and descending thoracic aorta (*DTA*) are controlled with red elastic vessel loops, a major collateral artery is controlled with a blue elastic vessel loop and the patent ductus arteriosus (*PDA*) is controlled with a black silk tie, **b** after occlusion of the proximal and the distal segments of the aortic isthmus with vascular clamps and resection of the narrowing, beginning of the end-to-end anastomosis of the posterior aortic wall with running suture, **c** the completed end-to-end anastomosis of the posterior aortic wall with running suture is shown, **d** the end-to-end anastomosis of the posterior aortic wall completed with interrupted sutures on the anterior aortic wall, **e** the final result after removal of the vascular clamps and, on the left side, the residual stump of the divided ductus arteriosus

▮ Surgical treatment

All these procedures are performed through a left postero-lateral thoracotomy without cardiopulmonary bypass. After longitudinal incision of the mediastinal pleura, the left subclavian artery, the descending thoracic aorta, the aortic arch and the collateral arteries are dissected free and controlled with elastic loops. If present, the patent ductus arteriosus is ligated and divided. The entire area of the isthmus is dissected free, and the vascular clamps chosen according to the preferred surgical option.

Occasionaly, in adults with complex anatomy or recurrent coarctation, a temporary bypass (from the ascending aorta or from the left atrium to the descending thoracic aorta) may be utilized.

In the case of repair of associated lesions with cardiopulmonary bypass from median sternotomy, the repair of aortic coarctation is performed through a transmediastinal approach.

▮ Resection and end-to-end anastomosis:
The standard procedure for discrete aortic coarctation: between two vascular clamps, the narrowed segment is incised widely enough to obtain an adequate aortic diameter both proximally and distally, and the two stumps are end-to-end anastomosed (Figs. 1.14.5 and 1.14.6); in neonates and/or in case of aortic arch hypoplasia this can be *extended* with an incision reaching the inferior aspect of the transverse aortic arch and with the distal segment of the descending thoracic aorta anastomosed to the undersurface of the aortic arch (Fig. 1.14.7); in adults, due to poor mobilization of the aortic stumps, *conduit interposition* may (rarely) be necessary after aortic resection in order to avoid excessive tension of the anastomosis (Fig. 1.14.8).

▮ Subclavian flap aortoplasty: The aortic enlargement is obtained by utilizing the left subclavian artery, divided before the ligated

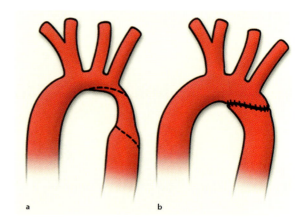

Fig. 1.14.7. Resection and end-to-end anastomosis extended to the aortic arch. **a** proximal incision reaching the inferior aspect of the transverse aortic arch, **b** end-to-end anastomosis completed with enlargement of the aortic arch

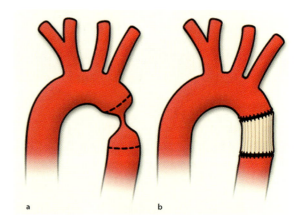

Fig. 1.14.8. Resection and end-to-end anastomosis with conduit interposition. **a** incisions proximally and distally to the long narrowing, **b** end-to-end anastomosis completed with conduit insertion

origin of the vertebral artery, and opened longitudinally; the incision is prolonged well below the aortic coarctation, and the coarctation shelf is carefully excised; the opened left subclavian artery is brought down and sutured to enlarge the aortic isthmus (Figs. 1.14.9 and 1.14.10); this can be modified into a *reverse subclavian flap* to enlarge a hypoplastic aortic arch.

▮ Patch aortoplasty: The aortic enlargement can be achieved with a biological (rare) or

Fig. 1.14.9. Subclavian flap aortoplasty. **a** division of the distal left subclavian artery and its incision prolonged well below the aortic coarctation, **b** wide opening of the left subclavian artery and of the aortic isthmus, after resection of the coarctation shelf, **c** completed anastomosis to enlarge the aortic isthmus with the opened left subclavian artery brought down and sutured as a flap

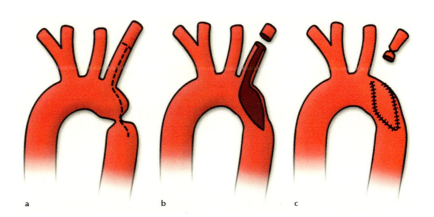

synthetic (frequent) patch, implanted to enlarge the narrow aortic isthmus, opened with a longitudinal incision (Fig. 1.14.11); despite the advantages of avoiding an extensive aortic dissection and mobilization as well as a circumferential suture line, this technique nowadays is virtually abandoned because of the frequent reports of aneurysm formation in the area of the prosthetic patch; an acceptable alternative option, particularly in infants, is aortoplasty using the enlarged base of the transected left subclavian artery.

▪ **Aortic bypass:** Rarely, in case of complex or recurrent coarctation or in case of pseudocoarctation (aortic kinking, without collateral circulation), a synthetic tubular pros-

thesis may be inserted between the ascending aorta (through an extended left or a right thoracotomy) or the left subclavian artery (left thoracotomy) and the distal descending thoracic aorta (Figs. 1.14.12 and 1.14.13).

▪ Potential complications

Residual or recurrent aortic coarctation, hemorrhage, paraplegia, paradoxical arterial hypertension, abdominal pain, mesentery (necrotising) vasculitis, chylothorax, aneurysm (after patch aortoplasty), left upper arm ischemia (after subclavian flap), recurrent nerve lesion.

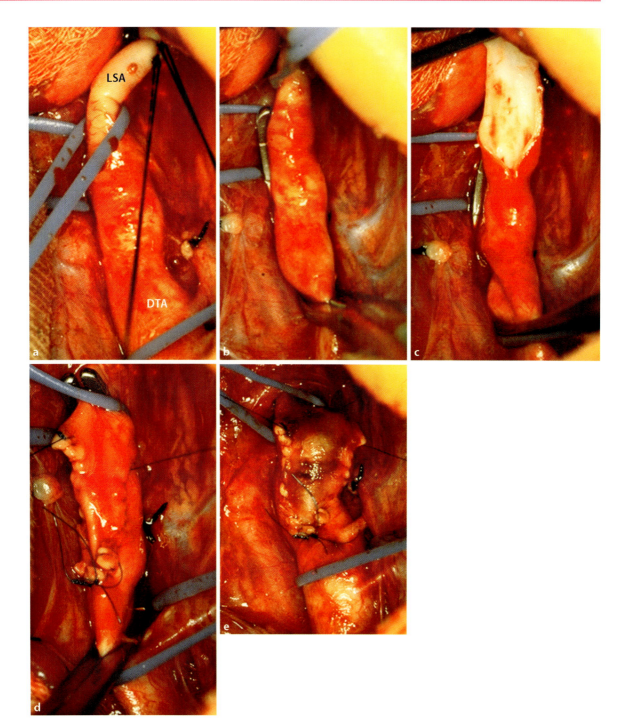

Fig. 1.14.10. Subclavian flap aortoplasty. **a** intra-operative photograph (postero-lateral left thoracotomy) showing the aortic arch, the left subclavian artery (*LSA*) and the descending thoracic aorta (*DTA*) controlled with blue elastic vessel loops; the distal end of the left subclavian artery and the origin of the left vertebral artery have already been ligated, **b** the aortic arch and the descending thoracic aorta controlled with a single vascular clamp, and the left subclavian artery controlled with a blue elastic vessel loop are shown, **c** the left subclavian artery, after distal division, opened with a longitudinal incision in direction of the aortic isthmus, **d** the completed anastomosis to enlarge the aortic isthmus with the opened left subclavian artery brought down and sutured as a flap is shown, **e** the final result after removal of the vascular clamp. The aortic arch and descending thoracic aorta are still controlled with blue elastic vessel loops

Fig. 1.14.11. Patch aortoplasty. **a** longitudinal incision across the narrowing, **b** wide opening of aortic isthmus, after resection of the coarctation shelf, **c** anastomosis of the prosthetic patch completed to enlarge the aortic isthmus

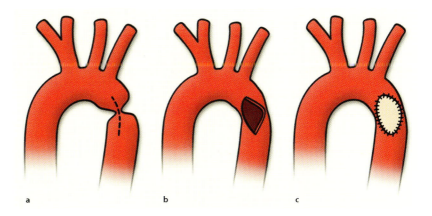

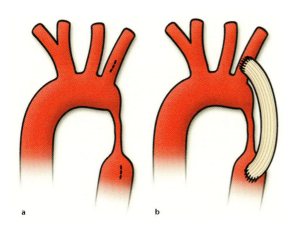

Fig. 1.14.12. Aortic bypass. **a** incisions on the left subclavian artery and on the descending thoracic aorta, proximally and distally to the obstruction, **b** aortic bypass completed with synthetic tubular prosthesis inserted between the left subclavian artery and the descending thoracic aorta

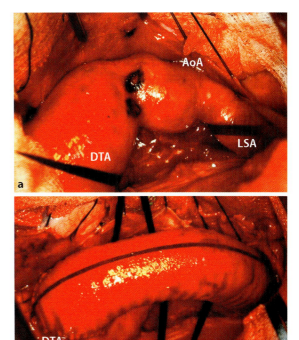

Fig. 1.14.13. Aortic bypass. **a** intra-operative photograph (postero-lateral left thoracotomy) showing the aortic pseudo-coarctation (aortic kinking, without collateral circulation); left subclavian artery (*LSA*) and descending thoracic aorta (*DTA*) are controlled with tapes (*AoA* aortic arch), **b** aortic bypass obtained with interposition of a tubular prosthesis between the left subclavian artery and descending thoracic aorta (*DTA*) is shown

▮ References

Brom AG (1965) Narrowing of the aortic isthmus and enlargement of the mind. J Thorac Cardiovasc Surg 50:166

Brouwer MHJ, Cromme-Dijkhuis AH, Ebels T, Eijgelaar A (1992) Growth of the hypoplastic aortic arch after simple coarctation resection and end-to-end anastomosis. J Thorac Cardiovasc Surg 104:426

Campbell M (1970) Natural history of coarctation of the aorta. Br Heart J 32:633

Celermajer DS, Greaves K (2002) Survivors of coarctation repair: fixed but not cured. Heart 88:113–114

Corno AF, Nijveld A, Schuller JL, Lam J, Bulterijs AHK, Marcelletti C (1982) Simplified thoracic approach to ascending and descending aorta for complex coarctation. Neth J Surg 34:27–30

Corno AF, Marcelletti C (1990) Bypass grafts for complex aortic coarctation: simplified approach. J Thorac Cardiovasc Surg 99:945–946

Corno AF (1993) Rare cardiac malformations. In: D'Alessandro LC (ed) Heart Surgery 1993. CESI, Rome, pp 189–199

Corno AF (2000) Surgery for congenital heart disease. Curr Opinion Cardiol 15:238–243

Corno AF, Botta U, Hurni M, Tozzi P, von Segesser LK (2001) Aortic coarctectomy in adults: 33-year experience. Med Cardiovasc 4:5S

Corno AF, Botta U, Hurni M, Galal OM, Payot M, Sekarski N, von Segesser LK (2001) Aortic coarctectomy in children: long-term single center observation. Cardiol Young 11(Suppl 1):159

Corno AF, Botta U, Hurni M, Payot M, Sekarski N, Tozzi P, von Segesser LK (2001) Surgery for aortic coarctation: a 30 years experience. Eur J Cardiothorac Surg 20:1202–1206

Crafoord C, Nylin G (1945) Congenital congenital of the aorta and its surgical treatment. J Thorac Surg 14:347

DeLeon SY, Idriss FS, Ilbawi MN, Tin N, Berry T (1981) Transmediastinal repair of complex coarctation and interrupted aortic arch. J Thorac Cardiovasc Surg 82:98

Del Nido PJ, Williams WG, Wilson GJ (1986) Synthetic patch angioplasty for repair of coarctation of the aorta: experience with aneurysm formation. Circulation 74(Suppl I):32–36

Downing DF, Grotzinger PJ, Weller RW (1958) Coarctation of the aorta. The syndrome of necrotizing arteritis of the small intestine following surgical therapy. Am J Dis Child 96:711

Edie RN, Janani J, Attai LA, Malm JR, Robinson G (1975) Bypass grafts for recurrent or complex coarctations of the aorta. Ann Thorac Surg 20:558

Elzenga NJ, Gittenberger-de-Groot AG (1983) Localized coarctation of the aorta: an age-dependent spectrum. Br Heart J 49:317–323

Ferencz C, Rubin JD, McCarter RJ (1985) Congenital heart disease: prevalence at livebirth. The Baltimore-Washington infant study. Am J Epidemiol 121:31–36

Fyler DC, Buckley LP, Hellenbrand WE, Cohn HE (1980) Report of the New England Regional Infant Care Program. Pediatrics 65 (Suppl):375–461

Giamberti A, Corno AF, Di Donato RM, Marianeschi SM, Amodeo A, Guccione P, Marcelletti C (1989) Coartazione aortica in etá pediatrica. Arch Chir Tor Cardiovasc 11:63

Gravante E, Iaquinta K, Fiorani A, Corno AF (1993) Assistenza ai pazienti con coartazione aortica. G Ital Cardiol 23 (Suppl 2):29

Gross RE (1945) Surgical correction for coarctation of the aorta. Surgery 18:673

Hart JC, Waldhausen JA (1983) Reversed subclavian flap angioplasty for arch coarctation of the aorta. Ann Thorac Surg 36:715

Hoffman JIE, Kaplan S (2002) The incidence of congenital heart disease. J Am Coll Cardiol 39:1890–1900

Lam J, Corno AF, Oorthuys HKE, Marcelletti C (1983) Unusual association of congenital heart disease in Noonan's syndrome. Pediatr Cardiol 3:23–26

Lisi G, Corno AF, Pierli C, Biagioli B, Santoro F, Sani G, De Giorgi L, Grossi A (1989) Aortic coarctation: surgery based on two-dimensional and Doppler echocardiography. Cuore 6:475–479

Marino B, Corno AF, Carotti A, Pasquini L, Giannico S, Guccione P, Bevilacqua M, De Simone G, Marcelletti C (1990) Pediatric cardiac surgery guided by echocardiography. Scand J Thorac Cardiovasc Surg 24:197–201

Nasser WK, Helmen C (1966) Kinking of the aortic arch (pseudocoarctation). Ann Intern Med 64:971

Papa M, Santoro F, Corno AF (1993) Spontaneous closure of inlet ventricular septal defect in an infant with Down's syndrome and aortic coarctation. Chest 104:620–622

Rudolph AM, Heymann MA, Spitznas U (1972) Hemodynamic considerations in the development of narrowing of the aorta. Am J Cardiol 30:514–525

Sade RM, Taylor AB, Chariker EP (1979) Aortoplasty compared with resection of the aorta in young children. Ann Thorac Surg 28:346–351

Sealy WC, Harris JS, Young WG, Calloway HA (1957) Paradoxical hypertension following resection of coarctation of the aorta. Surgery 42:135

Serfontein SJ, Kron IL (2002) Complications of coarctation repair. Semin Thorac Cardiovasc Surg 5:206–211

Swan L, Ashrafian H, Gatzoulis MA (2002) Repair of coarctation: a higher goal? Lancet 359:977–978

Vouhé PR, Trinquet F, Lecompte Y, Vernant F, Roux PM, Touati G, Pome G, Leca F, Neveux JY (1988) Aortic coarctation with hypoplastic aortic arch. Results of extended end-to-end aortic arch anastomosis. J Thorac Cardiovasc Surg 96:557

Waldhausen JA, Nohwald DL (1966) Repair of coarctation of the aorta with a subclavian flap. J Thorac Cardiovasc Surg 51:532–533

Incidence

Aortic arch interruption is the 20th most common congenital heart defect, representing a frequency of 0.003/1000 live births, and it accounts for 0.7% of congenital heart defects.

Morphology

The arch of the aorta is described as three segments: proximal, distal and isthmus. The proximal component extends from the take-off of the innominate artery to the left common carotid artery. The distal component extends from the left common carotid artery to the take-off of the left subclavian artery. The segment of aorta connecting the distal aortic arch to the juxtaductal region of the descending aorta is termed the isthmus. This complex composite of segments introduces a risk of developmental anomalies in the form of interruptions at the various junction points.

Aortic arch interruption is characterized by complete lack of anatomic continuity between the aortic arch or isthmus and the descending thoracic aorta. In aortic arch atresia, with identical pathophysiology and hemodynamics, there is anatomic continuity between the two segments, represented by an imperforate fibrous strand of various length.

Three anatomic types of aortic arch interruption have been described (Fig. 1.15.1):

- Type A: the interruption is distal to the left subclavian artery.
- Type B: the interruption is between the left common carotid artery and the left subclavian artery.
- Type C: the interruption is between the innominate artery and the left common carotid artery.

Associated anomalies

Patent ductus arteriosus, ventricular septal defect, actual or potential systemic left ventricular outflow tract obstruction, bicuspid aortic valve, double outlet right ventricle, univentricular heart with discordant ventriculo-arterial connection, aorto-pulmonary window, truncus arteriosus, atrial isomerism.

Patent ductus arteriosus is always present. The ventricular septal defect is nearly always present, in the majority of cases of malalignment-type, subpulmonic, because of posterior malalignment of the ventricular septum. Subaortic stenosis is also present, due to the posterior malalignment of the ventricular septum (Fig. 1.15.2).

Di George's syndrome. Absence or severe hypoplasia of the thymus is not uncommon in patients with interrupted aortic arch, especially those with type B interruption.

Pathophysiology

There may be little suspicion of serious heart disease during the early neonatal period until ductal closure begins. If this occurs

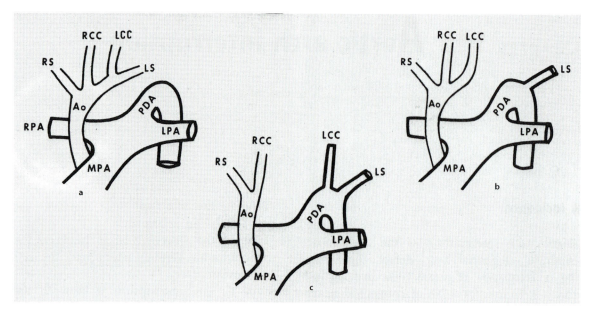

Fig. 1.15.1. Aortic arch interruption. The three anatomic types accordingly with the classification by Celoria and Patton (*Ao* ascending aorta, *LCC* left common carotid artery, *LPA* left pulmonary artery, *LS* left subclavian artery, *MPA* main pulmonary artery, *PDA* patent ductus arteriosus, *RCC* right common carotid artery, *RPA* right pulmonary artery, *RS* right subclavian artery) (reproduced with permission from Freedom RM, Benson LN, Smallhorn JF (1992) Neonatal heart disease. Springler, Berlin)

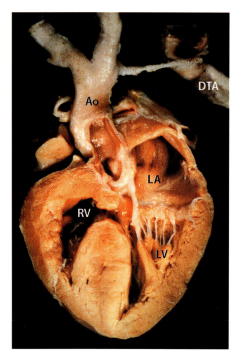

Fig. 1.15.2. Aortic arch interruption with ventricular septal defect of malalignment type and subaortic obstruction: morphology (*Ao* aorta, *DTA* descending thoracic aorta, *LA* left atrium, *LV* left ventricle, *RV* right ventricle) (photograph courtesy of Dr. Bruno Marino)

abruptly or is not recognized rapidly, the child will soon become profoundly acidotic and anuric as perfusion of the lower body becomes entirely dependent on collateral communication between the two separate aortic systems. Ischemic injury to the liver is reflected in a marked elevation of hepatic enzymes, and ischemic injury to the gut may be followed by evidence of necrotizing enterocolitis. Renal injury can be quantitated to some extent by the elevation observed in serum creatinine levels. Ultimately, a severe degree of systemic acidosis (prolonged pH less than 7.0) results in injury to all tissues of the body, including the brain and the heart itself. The child may have seizures and become flaccid and poorly responsive. Myocardial injury becomes apparent from decreased contractility and the low cardiac output state, despite normalization of other parameters. Because pulmonary blood flow is preserved during ductal closure, it is rare to see evidence of pulmonary insufficiency, although the child will hyperventilate in an attempt to compensate for the metabolic acidosis. Occasionally, the arterial duct does not close during the neonatal period, and the diagnosis may be delayed for several weeks. As pulmonary resistance falls, there will be an increasing left-to-right shunt, and the child will show evidence of congestive heart failure, including failure to thrive.

∎ Diagnosis

∎ **Clinical pattern:** almost all these neonates present with some respiratory distress, mild to severe cyanosis, varying degrees of congestive heart failure, and clinical evidence of low cardiac output; the distribution of palpable pulses depends on the anatomic subtype; cardiac examination demonstrates bulging left chest, hyperdynamic left precordium with prominent right ventricular impulse; the second sound is split, with systolic ejection murmur along the left sternal edge; gallop rhythm is frequent; the degree of liver enlargement reflects the severity of congestive heart failure.

∎ **Electrocardiogram:** frontal QRS axis to the right, with right ventricular hypertrophy and varying degrees of right or combined atrial enlargement.

∎ **Chest X-ray:** the cardiac imaging will depend upon the associated cardiac defects; cardiomegaly and increased pulmonary markings are common.

∎ **Echocardiogram:** an accurate anatomic diagnosis can be made with echocardiography alone; this is an important advantage to the critically ill neonate, because the additional insult of an invasive cardiac catheterization can be avoided; in addition to localizing the site of the interruption, echocardiography should provide the following information:
- the distance between the discontinuous aortic segments,
- the narrowest dimension of the left ventricular outflow tract (generally related to posterior displacement of the infundib-

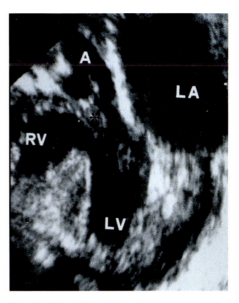

Fig. 1.15.3. Echocardiography: parasternal long-axis view showing the ventricular septal defect of malalignment type with subaortic obstruction (*A* aorta, *LA* left atrium, *LV* left ventricle, *RV* right ventricle, *** = malaligned infundibular septum) (reproduced with permission from Marino B, Thiene G (1990) Atlante di anatomia ecocardiografica delle cardiopatie congenite, USES, Firenze)

ular septum), the diameter of the aortic annulus, and the diameter of the ascending aorta,
- the features of associated anomalies (Fig. 1.15.3).

∎ **Cardiac catheterization:** because the diagnosis is generally made when ductal patency has been re-established using PGE$_1$ (Fig. 1.15.4), pressure data are of little use in formulating a plan for surgical management; there are left-to-right shunt at the atrial and ventricular levels, pulmonary artery and right ventricular systemic pressure, elevated end-diastolic pressures in both ventricles; the issue that most commonly arises concerns the adequacy of the left ventricular outflow tract: attempts to quantitate the degree of obstruction by measuring a pressure gradient are hampered by the left ventricular decompression through the ventricular septal defect, almost always nonrestrictive; there is no evidence that multiple ventricular septal

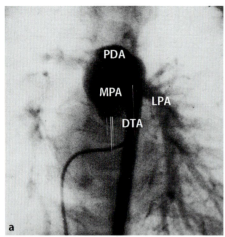

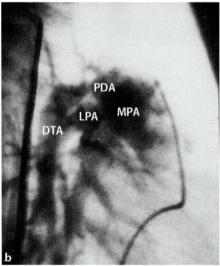

Fig. 1.15.4. Aortic arch interruption: angiography. **a** antero-posterior view: contrast injection in the main pulmonary artery, with subsequent opacification of the descending thoracic aorta via the patent ductus arteriosus, **b** lateral view: contrast injection in the main pulmonary artery, with subsequent opacification of the descending thoracic aorta via the patent ductus arteriosus (*DTA* descending thoracic aorta, *LPA* left pulmonary artery, *MPA* main pulmonary artery, *PDA* patent ductus arteriosus)

defects are more accurately identified by angiography than by echocardiography.

▮ Indications for surgical treatment

PGE_1 has revolutionized the management of interrupted aortic arch. Establishing ductal patency represents just the first step in medical resuscitation of the neonate with an in-terrupted aortic arch. Because the lower half of the body is dependent on perfusion through the arterial duct and because blood in the arterial duct has the choice of passing into the pulmonary or the systemic circulation, it is important to maximize the pulmonary vascular resistance. This can be achieved by avoiding an elevated FiO_2 and by avoiding respiratory alkalosis through hyperventilation. In fact, control of ventilation is best accomplished by intubating the neonate, sedating him or her with a fentanyl infusion, and inducing paralysis with pancuronium. A peak inspiratory pressure and ventilatory rate that will achieve a PCO_2 level of 40 to 60 mmHg should be selected. Metabolic acidosis must be aggressively treated with intravenous administration of sodium bicarbonate. Because myocardial function is likely to be depressed and because it may be necessary for the heart to handle a moderate to severe volume load, an inotropic agent such as dopamine is employed. Dopamine has the advantage of maximizing renal perfusion in a context of an ischemic renal injury. Complete resuscitation should be achieved before operative intervention is undertaken, since this approach resulted in a significant improvement in surgical outcome. It is wrong to take a child to the operating room with any acid-base, renal, or hepatic abnormalities.

The diagnosis alone is the indication for surgery.

▮ Surgical treatment

Two surgical approaches are available: a) two-stages, with repair of the interrupted aortic arch (direct anastomosis of the proximal and distal aortic segments after extensive mobilization) through a left postero-lateral thoracotomy, with or without pulmonary artery banding, followed by median sternotomy to close the ventricular septal defect; b) single stage, through median sternotomy (Fig. 1.15.5), with simultaneous repair of the interrupted aortic arch and patch

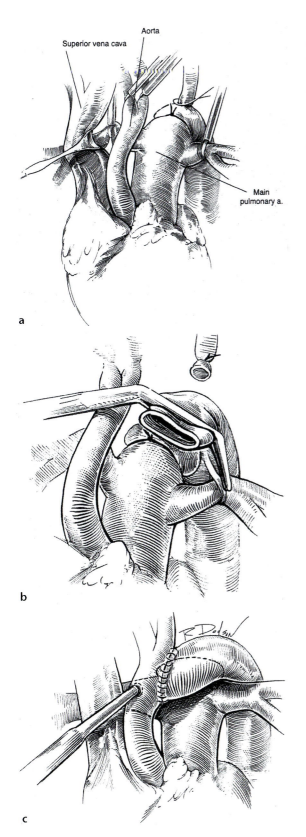

Superior vena cava

Aorta

Main pulmonary a.

a

b

R Dodson

c

closure of the ventricular septal defect on cardiopulmonary bypass. The choice is dictated by the presence of associated lesions, in particular by the presence of severe left ventricular outflow tract obstruction.

In the absence of associated lesions other than patent ductus arteriosus and ventricular septal defect, primary repair by direct anastomosis of the arch with closure of the ventricular septal defect is the preferred surgical approach. The main reason is that pulmonary artery banding might promote or aggravate subaortic stenosis in patients with a malalignment ventricular septal defect. Although the primary repair is physiologically corrective, it should not be viewed as fully curative due to the high incidence of significant late obstruction of the left ventricular outflow tract.

Left ventricular outflow tract obstruction. The morphology of left ventricular outflow tract obstruction with interrupted aortic arch varies, and therefore, surgical management also varies according to the specific circumstances. In some cases it is possible to resect the posteriorly deviated infundibular septum through the aortic valve. An aortic valvotomy may also be required if there is aortic valve stenosis. If there is annular hypoplasia with a long tunnel subaortic stenosis, the approach is to perform an annular enlarging procedure such as the extended aortic root replacement, with either a posterior incision into the anterior leaflet of the mitral valve (for less severe stenosis) or an

Fig. 1.15.5. Surgical treatment. **a** surgical approach from median sternotomy, with dissection of both pulmonary arteries and the neck vessels, all controlled with snares, **b** after extensive mobilization, the descending thoracic aorta, controlled with a vascular clamp, is pulled anteriorly to reach the ascending aorta, **c** with a period of deep hypothermia and circulatory arrest, the descending thoracic aorta is end-to-side anastomosed to the ascending aorta; the aortic cannula is then introduced in the ascending aorta for reperfusion and rewarming (reproduced with permission from Castaneda AR, Jonas RA, Mayer JE, Hanley FL (1994) Cardiac surgery of the neonate and infant. WB Saunders Company, Philadelphia)

anterior incision into the ventricular septum (for very severe stenosis). In the presence of an unfavorable ratio (<0.6) of the left ventricular outflow tract to the ascending aorta diameter, a univentricular type of approach (Norwood) is advised.

▮ Potential complications

Residual pressure gradient at the level of the aortic arch anastomosis and/or at the left ventricular outflow tract, residual ventricular septal defect, complete atrio-ventricular block, left bronchial obstruction.

▮ **Left bronchial obstruction:** The left main bronchus passes under the aortic arch. If a direct anastomosis is performed without adequate mobilization of the ascending and descending aorta, a bowstring effect over the left main bronchus may result. This is manifested by air trapping in the left lung with hyperexpansion, as seen on chest radiography and confirmed by bronchoscopy. Surgical management may require an ascending-to-descending aortic conduit after division of the arch.

▮ **Di George's syndrome:** The long-term immune status of survivors after surgery for aortic arch interruption requires further assessment and follow up.

▮ References

Barrat-Boyes BG, Nicholls TT, Brandt PWT, Neutze JM (1972) Aortic arch interruption associated with patent ductus arteriosus, ventricular septal defect, and total anomalous pulmonary venous connection. J Thorac Cardiovasc Surg 63:367

Bogers AJ, Contant CM, Hokken RB, Cromme-Dijkhuis AH (1997) Repair of aortic arch interruption by direct anastomosis. Eur J Cardiothorac Surg 11:100–104

Bruins C (1978) Competition between aortic isthmus and ductus arteriosus: reciprocal influence of structure and flow. Eur J Cardiol 8:87–97

Celoria GC, Patton RB (1959) Congenital absence of the aortic arch. Am Heart J 58:407–413

Corno AF, Lam J, Becker AE, Marcelletti C (1981) Aortic arch interruption. G Ital Cardiol 11:679–685

DeLeon SY, Idriss FS, Ilbawi MN, Tin N, Berry T (1981) Transmediastinal repair of complex coarctation and interrupted aortic arch. J Thorac Cardiovasc Surg 82:98

Freedom RM, Bain HH, Esplugas E, Dische R, Rowe RD (1977) Ventricular septal defect in interruption of aortic arch. Am J Cardiol 39:572–582

Ferencz C, Rubin JD, McCarter RJ (1985) Congenital heart disease: prevalence at livebirth. The Baltimore-Washington infant study. Am J Epidemiol 121:31–36

Foker JE (1992) Surgical repair of aortic arch interruption. Ann Thorac Surg 53:369–370

Fyler DC, Buckley LP, Hellenbrand WE, Cohn HE (1980) Report of the New England Regional Infant Care Program. Pediatrics 65 (Suppl):375–461

Ho SY, Wilcox BR, Anderson RH, Lincoln JCR (1983) Interrupted aortic arch: anatomical features of surgical significance. J Thorac Cardiovasc Surg 31:199–205

Karl TR, Sano S, Brawn W, Mee RBB (1992) Repair of hypoplastic or interrupted aortic arch via sternotomy. J Thorac Cardiovasc Surg 103:866

Luciani GB, Ackerman RJ, Chang AC, Wells WJ, Starnes VA (1996) One-stage repair of interrupted aortic arch, ventricular septal defect, and subaortic obstruction in the neonate: a novel approach. J Thorac Cardiovasc Surg 111:348–358

Monro JL, Delany DJ, Ogilvie BC, Salmon AP, Keeton BR (1996) Growth potential in the new aortic arch after non-end-to-end repair of aortic arch interruption in infancy. Ann Thorac Surg 61:1212–1216

Roberts WC, Morrow AG, Braunwald E (1962) Complete interruption of the aortic arch. Circulation 26:39

Roussin R, Belli E, Lacour-Gayet F, Godart F, Rey C, Bruniaux J, Planché C, Serraf A (2002) Aortic arch reconstruction with pulmonary autograft patch aortoplasty. J Thorac Cardiovasc Surg 123:443–448

Rudolph AM, Heymann MA, Spitznas U (1972) Hemodynamic considerations in the development of narrowing of the aorta. Am J Cardiol 30:514–525

Sell JE, Jonas RA, Mayer JE, Blackstone EH, Kirklin JW, Castaneda AR (1988) The results of a surgical program for interrupted aortic arch. J Thorac Cardiovasc Surg 96:864–877

Trusler GA, Izukawa T (1975) Interrupted aortic arch and ventricular septal defect. Direct repair through a median sternotomy incision in a 13-day old infant. J Thorac Cardiovasc Surg 69:126

CHAPTER 1.16 Complete transposition of the great arteries

▌ Incidence

Complete transposition of the great arteries is the 6th most common congenital heart defect (4.7% of all congenital heart defects), and the second most common congenital heart disease encountered in early infancy, for 0.2–0.4/1000 of live births. It is also the most common cause of transfer to the cardiac care in neonates. Transposition of the great arteries is more frequent in males.

▌ Morphology (Figs. 1.16.1 and 1.16.2)

Transposition of the great arteries is an abnormality of ventriculo-arterial connection, with the aorta originating from the morphologically right ventricle and the pulmonary artery from the morphologically left ventricle.

The aorta is anterior and slightly to the right of the main pulmonary artery (Fig. 1.16.3). The aortic valve is to the right of the pulmonary valve but still anterior to it. The main pulmonary artery is in such a position with the left ventricle, thus, allowing direct flow into the right pulmonary artery; as a consequence the right pulmonary artery becomes larger, with more flow to the right lung.

There are four major subgroups of complete transposition of the great arteries:

▐ Transposition of the great arteries with intact ventricular septum (Fig. 1.16.4) or with restrictive ventricular septal defect (60% of the cases).

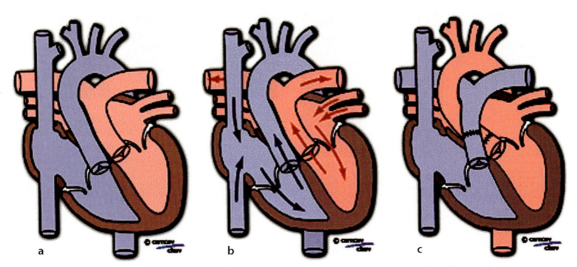

Fig. 1.16.1. Transposition of the great arteries with intact ventricular septum: **a** morphology, **b** pathophysiology, **c** surgery

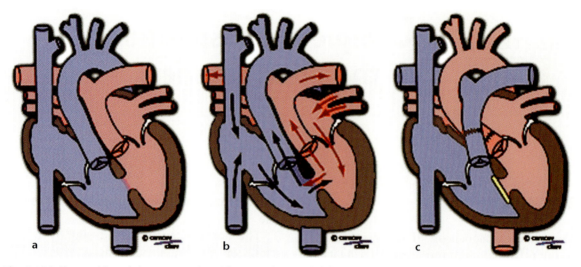

Fig. 1.16.2. Transposition of the great arteries with ventricular septal defect: **a** morphology, **b** pathophysiology, **c** surgery

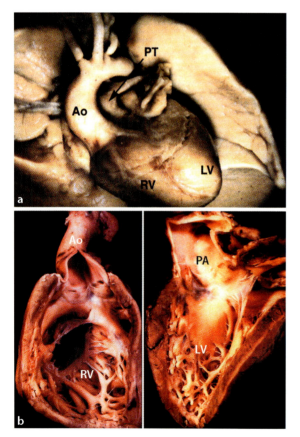

Fig. 1.16.3. Transposition of the great arteries: morphology. **a** external appearance, with the aorta anterior and slightly to the right of the main pulmonary artery, **b** internal appearance, with abnormality of ventriculo-arterial connection: aorta originating from the morphologically right ventricle and pulmonary artery from the morphologically left ventricle (*Ao* aorta, *LV* left ventricle, *PA* pulmonary artery, *PT* pulmonary artery trunk, *RV* right ventricle) (photographs courtesy of Dr. Enrico Chiappa)

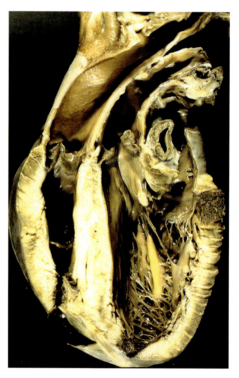

Fig. 1.16.4. Transposition of the great arteries: morphology. Transposition of the great arteries with intact ventricular septum (reproduced with permission from Marino B, Thiene G (1990) Atlante di anatomia ecocardiografica delle cardiopatie congenite, USES, Firenze)

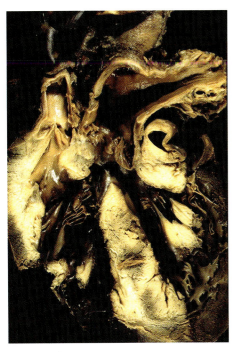

Fig. 1.16.5. Transposition of the great arteries: morphology. Transposition of the great arteries with ventricular septal defect (photograph courtesy of Dr. Bruno Marino)

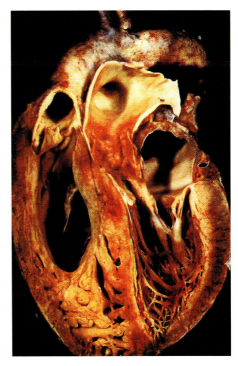

Fig. 1.16.7. Transposition of the great arteries: morphology. Transposition of the great arteries with intact ventricular septum and left ventricular outflow tract obstruction (photograph courtesy of Dr. Enrico Chiappa)

■ Transposition of the great arteries with unrestrictive ventricular septal defect (Fig. 1.16.5) (20%).

■ Transposition of the great arteries with ventricular septal defect and left ventricular outflow tract obstruction (15%) (Fig. 1.16.6).

■ Transposition of the great arteries with intact ventricular septum and left ventricular outflow tract obstruction (5%) (Fig. 1.16.7).

■ Associated anomalies

Most infants with complete transposition of the great arteries have patent foramen ovale and a patent ductus arteriosus.

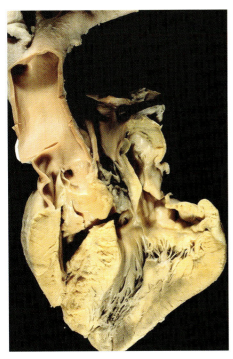

Fig. 1.16.6. Transposition of the great arteries: morphology. Transposition of the great arteries with ventricular septal defect and left ventricular outflow tract obstruction (photograph courtesy of Dr. Bruno Marino)

■ **Ventricular septal defect:** Fifty percent (50%) of patients with transposition of the great arteries have ventricular septal defects. One-third of patients with complete transposition of the great arteries and ventricular septal defect will have closure of the ventricular septal defect in the first year of life.

The most common position of ventricular septal defects in transposition of the great arteries is the infundibular septum, with or without malalignment, followed by defects in the membranous septum.

▮ Left ventricular outflow tract obstruction (=pulmonary stenosis):

After ventricular septal defect, left ventricular outflow tract obstruction is the most commonly associated cardiac defect with transposition of the great arteries (25–30%).

Pulmonary stenosis (left ventricular outflow tract obstruction) in patients with transposition of the great arteries is due to the leftward bowing of the ventricular septum due to the elevated (systemic) right ventricular pressure, and to the close proximity of the mitral valve to the ventricular septum, leading to dynamic obstruction. Anatomical valvular or subvalvular pulmonary stenosis are more rare, and mainly due to tissue tags, aneurysm of the membranous septum, straddling of the atrio-ventricular valve or pulmonary valve stenosis.

▮ Coronary arteries
(Fig. 1.16.8): In 60% of patients, the right coronary artery originates from the right coronary sinus and the left coronary artery, which gives origin to the circumflex and left anterior descending, from the left coronary sinus.

In 10% of patients, the right coronary artery and the circumflex originate from the right coronary sinus with the left anterior descending originating from the left coronary sinus. In these cases the circumflex is located posteriorly to the pulmonary artery.

In another 10% of the patients, the circumflex originates from the right coronary sinus and the right coronary artery and left anterior descending originate from the left coronary sinus (Fig. 1.16.9). In these cases the right coronary artery is located rightwards anterior to the aorta.

In another 10% of patients, the right coronary artery originates from the right coronary sinus and gives origin to the right coronary artery and the left coronary artery. In these cases the left coronary artery is located in between the aorta and the pulmonary artery and gives origin to the circumflex and the left anterior descending branches.

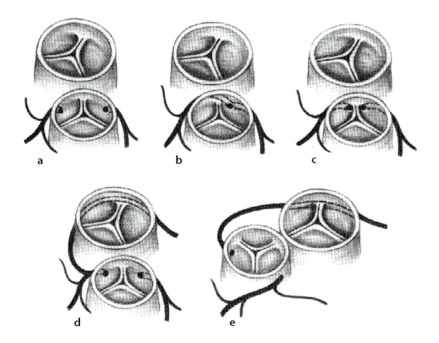

Fig. 1.16.8. Transposition of the great arteries: coronary arteries. Yacoub and Radley-Smith classification of the anatomy of the coronary arteries in transposition of the great arteries (reproduced with permission from Yacoub MH, Radley-Smith R (1978) Anatomy of the coronary arteries in transposition of the great arteries and methods for their transfer in anatomical correction. Thorax 33:418–424)

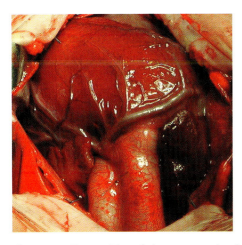

Fig. 1.16.9. Transposition of the great arteries. Intra-operative photograph showing transposition of the great arteries with the right coronary artery and left anterior descending coronary artery originating from the left coronary sinus (photograph courtesy of Dr. Piero Abbruzzese)

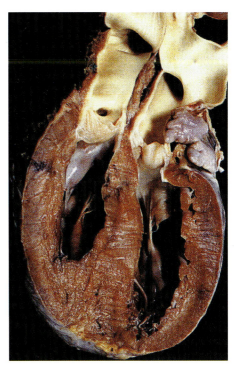

Fig. 1.16.10. Transposition of the great arteries: left juxtaposition of the auricular appendages (photograph courtesy of Dr. Enrico Chiappa)

In 5% of patients, there is a single origin of all the coronary arteries, either from the right or from the left sinus, and this anomaly can complicate the surgical technique of arterial switch.

The most troublesome coronary anomaly, in view of an arterial switch, is the presence of an intramural coronary artery (3–5%): in this situation the first portion of a coronary artery, generally the left, is located within the aortic wall, before assuming epicardial distribution.

■ **Other associated anomalies:** Right aortic arch is seen in 4% of patients with intact ventricular septum and in 8% of patients with ventricular septal defect. Right aortic arch is more common (10%) in patients with transposition of the great arteries with pulmonary stenosis or pulmonary atresia.

Other associated anomalies include the following: aortic coarctation (5%), left juxtaposition of the auricular appendages (2–4%) (Fig. 1.16.10), malformations of the tricuspid (including Ebstein's anomaly) or the mitral valve, right or left ventricular hypoplasia, supero-inferior ventricles, subaortic stenosis.

■ Pathophysiology

The systemic and pulmonary circulations are in parallel (Fig. 1.16.11), instead of being in series as in normal hearts. Survival depends upon adequate communication between the two circulations, in order to allow for adequate *mixing* of oxygenated and desaturated blood. The most effective *mixing* occurs at the atrial level, because the communication is between the two low pressure chambers.

In order to understand the pathophysiology of complete transposition of the great arteries, it is necessary to understand the concept of *effective pulmonary blood flow*. The amount of oxygen taken up in the lungs depends upon the *effective pulmonary blood* flow, the amount of desaturated blood which comes from the systemic venous return (venae cavae and coronary sinus) reaches the pulmonary circulation. In normal hearts, without intra-cardiac shunt, the *effective pulmonary blood flow* is equal to the *total pul-*

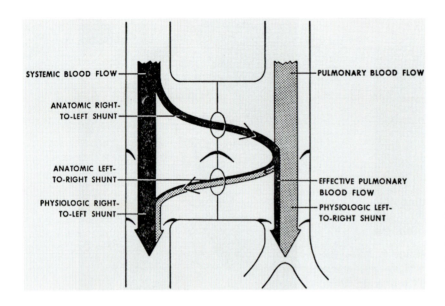

Fig. 1.16.11. Transposition of the great arteries: pathophysiology (reproduced with permission from Rudolph AM (2001) Congenital diseases of the heart: clinical-physiological considerations. Futura Publishing Company, Armonk)

monary blood flow, which in fact reflects the systemic venous return. In complete transposition of the great arteries the *effective pulmonary blood flow*, and therefore the level of systemic oxygenation, depends upon the extent of *mixing* between systemic and pulmonary circulations, as represented by the anatomic right-to-left and left-to-right shunts. In this situation with parallel circulations, the absolute amounts of shunt in either direction are equal.

Despite a large *total pulmonary blood flow*, in the presence of a little *mixing* at the atrial level, the systemic arterial saturation will remain low; while with adequate *mixing* at atrial level, the *total pulmonary blood flow* will influence the arterial oxygen saturation.

In the presence of adequate *mixing* at the atrial level, the systemic arterial saturation depends upon the ratio between the systemic and pulmonary blood flows.

Therefore, severe hypoxia is the result of either inadequate *mixing* at atrial level and/ or severe reduction of the *total pulmonary blood flow* (severe left ventricular outflow tract obstruction or increased pulmonary vascular resistance).

Patients with an intact ventricular septum tend to have dynamic left ventricular outflow tract obstruction, usually reversible after atrial or arterial switch operation.

Patients with an anatomic left ventricular outflow tract obstruction tend to have better left-to-right shunting in the ventricular septal defect and less cyanosis than others.

Patients with ventricular septal defects tend to have better mixing of the pulmonary and systemic circulations, but may become more cyanotic as the ventricular septal defect becomes smaller.

■ Diagnosis

■ **Clinical pattern:** the neonates are typically full term; neonates with transposition of the great arteries and intact ventricular septum or very small ventricular septal defect present early in the first day or two of life with cyanosis not improving with oxygen therapy; neonates with a ventricular septal defect present with cyanosis and congestive heart failure typically at a later date; these patients are typically tachypneic and cyanotic; on auscultation there is a single second heart sound; a murmur is heard in patients with a ventricular septal defect; in addition, left ventricular outflow tract obstruction may cause systolic ejection murmur.

■ **Electrocardiogram:** when performed early, the heart is within normal limits and later

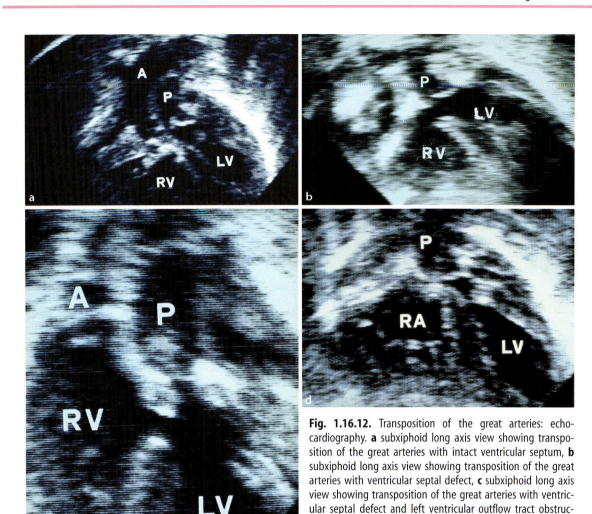

Fig. 1.16.12. Transposition of the great arteries: echocardiography. **a** subxiphoid long axis view showing transposition of the great arteries with intact ventricular septum, **b** subxiphoid long axis view showing transposition of the great arteries with ventricular septal defect, **c** subxiphoid long axis view showing transposition of the great arteries with ventricular septal defect and left ventricular outflow tract obstruction, **d** subxiphoid long axis view showing transposition of the great arteries with intact ventricular septum and left ventricular outflow tract obstruction (*A* aorta, *LV* left ventricle, *P* pulmonary artery, *RV* right ventricle) (reproduced with permission from Marino B, Thiene G (1990) Atlante di anatomia ecocardiografica delle cardiopatie congenite, USES, Firenze)

will show right ventricular hypertrophy; if left ventricular hypertrophy is present with left axis deviation then straddling of the tricuspid valve or overriding with right ventricular hyperplasia should be suspected.

▪ **Chest X-ray:** early on, the heart is also within normal limits, but later, particularly in patients with ventricular septal defect, cardiomegaly and increased pulmonary blood flow will develop; at a later age, the heart will present in the typical egg-on-side shape: this is because of biventricular dilatation and narrow mediastinum due to the positions of the great arteries.

▪ **Echocardiogram:** echocardiography demonstrates the anatomy (Fig. 1.16.12); the following particular features should be assessed:
– ventricular septal defect, its site and size,
– patent foramen ovale or atrial septal defect,
– patent ductus arteriosus,
– anatomy of the coronary arteries,
– aortic arch and its orientation,
– left ventricular outflow tract and presence of any obstruction, dynamic or anatomic,
– right ventricular size and function.

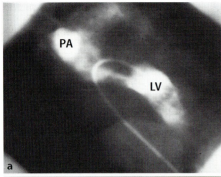

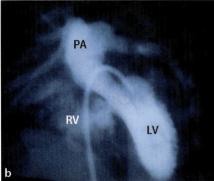

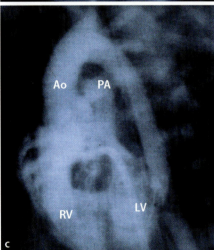

Fig. 1.16.13. Transposition of the great arteries: angio-cardiography. **a** left ventricular injection showing transposition of the great arteries with intact ventricular septum, **b** left ventricular injection showing transposition of the great arteries with ventricular septal defect, **c** left ventricular injection showing transposition of the great arteries with multiple ventricular septal defects (*Ao* aorta, *LV* left ventricle, *PA* pulmonary artery, *RV* right ventricle)

■ **Cardiac catheterization:** cardiac catheterization with angiography (Fig. 1.16.13) is indicated when:

– the coronary artery anatomy is not clear,
– the left ventricular outflow tract obstruction is thought to be anatomic rather than dynamic,
– a Rashkind balloon atrio-septostomy (Fig. 1.16.14) is needed, although this can be performed under echocardiographic guidance.

■ Indications for surgical treatment

■ **Transposition of the great arteries with intact ventricular septum or with restrictive ventricular septal defect:** There are two potential options for surgical repair: atrial rerouting (Mustard or Senning operation) and arterial switch (Jatene operation).

Atrial rerouting has been extensively utilized in the past, because of the following reasons:

■ after an adequate Rashkind balloon atrio-septostomy, in the presence of adequate oxygenation it was possible to delay the surgical repair for several months, reaching an age and a body weight better suitable to tolerate intra-cardiac repair;

■ it was a relatively simple procedure, with acceptable early and long-term results. Of course the draw-back of the atrial rerouting was the fact that right ventricle and tricuspid valve were left to substain lifelong systemic pressure lifelong, and this is accompanied by an increasing incidence over the years of right ventricular dysfunction and/or tricuspid valve regurgitation.

Since left ventricle and mitral valve are better suited to be the systemic ventricle and systemic atrio-ventricular valve, the arterial switch operation is therefore considered the best option for surgical repair. Patients with transposition of the great arteries with intact ventricular septum are best repaired 1–2 weeks after birth, because a drop in the pul-

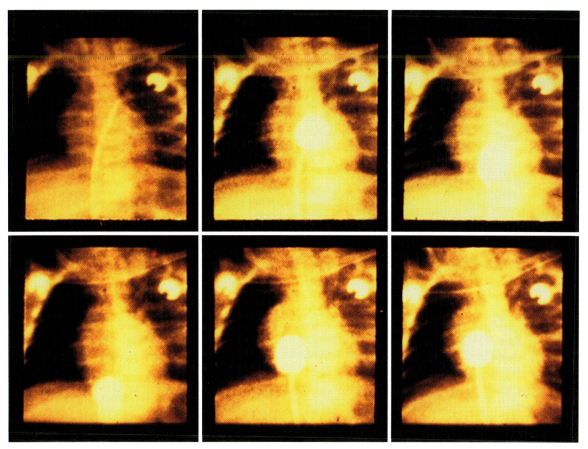

Fig. 1.16.14. Transposition of the great arteries: angiocardiography. Sequence of a Rashkind balloon atrio-septostomy

monary vascular resistance will cause deconditioning of the left ventricle, making repair with an arterial switch poorly tolerated at that point.

The left ventricle should be at or close to the systemic pressure to withstand becoming the systemic ventricle after the arterial switch operation.

For infants with transposition of the great arteries with an intact ventricular septum, with an arterial switch performed after 2 weeks of age but within the first 2–3 months of age, there is an increasing risk that they will require a period of mechanical circulatory assistance after surgery, in order to allow for adaptation of the left ventricle to substain the systemic circulation.

Whenever the patients are referred too late (after 2–3 months of age) for an arterial switch, there are two possibilities: either an atrial rerouting (Mustard or Senning operation) is considered, or the arterial switch needs to be preceeded by a left ventricular retraining: this is obtained by a pulmonary artery banding (to increase the left ventricular mass), associated with a systemic-to-pulmonary artery shunt (to increase the *total pulmonary blood flow* in order to tolerate the reduced oxygenation) and/or atrio-septectomy (to improve the *mixing* at atrial level in the case of restrictive interatrial communication) (Fig. 1.16.15).

■ **Transposition of the great arteries with an unrestrictive ventricular septal defect:** Atrial rerouting and closure of the ventricular septal defect has been practically abandoned, because the long-term complications of the atrial rerouting are much more frequent and severe than with atrial rerouting alone.

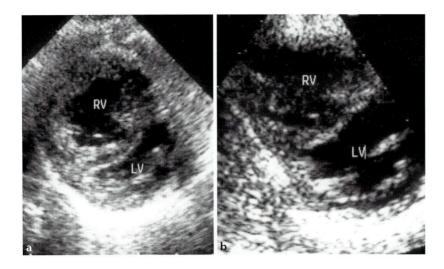

Fig. 1.16.15. Transposition of the great arteries. Echocardiography showing the right/left ventricular ratio before (**a**) and after (**b**) left ventricular retraining (pulmonary artery banding, systemic-to-pulmonary artery shunt and atrio-septectomy) after an interval of 6 months; the left ventricular retraining was followed by successful arterial switch

Therefore, since the left ventricle is better suited to be the systemic ventricle, the arterial switch operation with closure of the ventricular septal defect is the option of choice. This is generally done in infants with transposition of the great arteries and ventricular septal defect within the first 2–3 months of age; because of the presence of an unrestrictive ventricular septal defect, the left ventricle remains at systemic pressure and it can withstand becoming the systemic ventricle after the arterial switch operation.

Palliation with pulmonary artery banding can be utilized in infants with multiple ventricular septal defects.

■ Transposition of the great arteries with a ventricular septal defect and left ventricular outflow tract obstruction:

In infancy, patients with significant left ventricular outflow tract obstruction (anatomic) with ventricular septal defect are treated by a palliative procedure (systemic-to-pulmonary artery shunt) in order to increase the *total pulmonary blood flow* and reduce the cyanosis.

Surgical repair is performed generally after 1–2 years of age with a Rastelli procedure (closure of ventricular septal defect by creating a tunnel connecting the left ventricle to the aorta, and continuity between right ventricle and pulmonary artery obtained with a biological valved conduit) or a Lecompte procedure (or REV = Réparation à

l'Etage Ventriculaire: connection of the left ventricle to the aorta by closure of ventricular septal defect with a straight patch after infundibular resection, and direct implantation of the transected pulmonary artery on the right ventricle).

In cases with side-by-side great arteries or with intramural coronary arteries, an alternative surgical option, very rarely used, is the Damus-Kaye-Stansel procedure (arterial repair without coronary artery relocation).

■ Transposition of the great arteries with intact ventricular septum and left ventricular outflow tract obstruction:

These patients are very cyanotic early in life, and therefore they require an unrestrictive interatrial communication in order to maximize the *mixing* at the atrial level. However, very rarely, an additional systemic-to-pulmonary shunt is required.

If the left ventricular outflow tract obstruction is only dynamic and severe enough to maintain systemic pressure in the left ventricle, an arterial switch operation is feasible; the degree of the left ventricular outflow tract obstruction generally diminish after surgery.

Infants with anatomical left ventricular outflow tract obstruction can benefit from atrial rerouting and resection of the fibromuscular left ventricular outflow tract or implantation of a left ventricle to pulmonary artery valved conduit.

▪ **Other situations with associated anomalies:** Transposition of the great arteries with coarctation of the aorta is rare and usually associated with ventricular septal defect. There is an increased *total pulmonary blood flow* due to the high systemic vascular resistance secondary to the coarctation, resulting in congestive heart failure. Surgical management can be staged by fixing the coarctation first (with or without an associated pulmonary artery banding) and then performing an arterial switch operation, or total surgical repair (aortic coarctectomy and arterial switch) can be performed in a single stage.

Patients with severe right ventricular hypoplasia and tricuspid valve anomalies are better candidates for a univentricular type of repair (cavo-pulmonary connection).

Palliative atrial rerouting or arterial switch can be performed in patients with transposition of the great arteries with ventricular septal defect and pulmonary vascular obstructive disease to reduce cyanosis. In patients with transposition of the great arteries with intact ventricular septum and pulmonary vascular obstructive disease, palliative atrial rerouting is associated with the creation of a ventricular septal defect.

Conversion of a failing atrial rerouting to an arterial switch procedure requires that the pulmonary artery banding is performed first for a period of time until the left ventricle is able to tolerate the systemic pressure.

▪ **Surgical treatment (on cardiopulmonary bypass)**

▪ **Atrioseptectomy:** The original procedure of atrioseptectomy (Blalock-Hanlon), now virtually abandoned, is performed without cardiopulmonary bypass. Through a right anterior thoracotomy, after antephrenic pericardial opening, the right pulmonary artery and veins are temporary occluded. With a partial occluding clamp excluding each portion of the right and left atrial wall and the relative interatrial septum, through two parallel incisions on each atrial wall the lateral portion of the interatrial septum is excised. The edges of the two atrial incisions are then sutured together, leaving an unrestricted interatrial communication.

▪ **Atrial rerouting:** *Mustard procedure* (Fig. 1.16.16): After a longitudinal right atriotomy, the atrial septum is excised and the raw margins oversewn. The roof of the coronary sinus is incised. A pre-measured patch of autologous or heterologous pericardium or prosthetic material (Teflon, PTFE) is sutured in a way to reroute the systemic venous return from the superior and inferior vena cava to the mitral valve and therefore left ventricle and pulmonary artery. The right atriotomy is then closed with a pericardial (or PTFE) patch enlarging the new pulmonary venous channel, where the pulmonary venous return is rerouted to the tricuspid valve and therefore right ventricle and aorta.

Senning procedure (Fig. 1.16.17): After right atriotomy, the atrial septum is incised to create a flap, together with the lateral right atrial wall, in a way so as to reroute the systemic venous return from superior and inferior vena cava to the mitral valve and therefore left ventricle and pulmonary artery. The pulmonary venous channel is completed by suturing the anterior edge of the right atrial incision to the lateral edge of the left atrial incision.

▪ **Arterial switch (Jatene operation)** (Fig. 1.16.18): Aorta and pulmonary artery are transected above the sinuses. The coronary arteries are excised from the aortic root with a botton of aorta and implanted in the new aortic root (old pulmonary artery). The pulmonary artery bifurcation is brought anteriorly to the aorta (*Lecompte maneuver*) and the ascending aorta is anastomosed to the new aortic root. A portion of pericardium is utilized to close the defects created in the neo-pulmonary root (old aorta) by the excision of the coronary arteries, and the pulmonary artery bifurcation is anastomosed to the new pulmonary artery root.

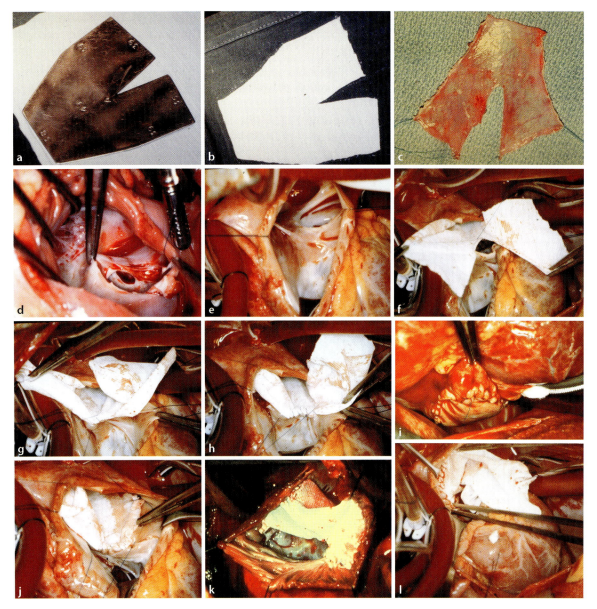

Fig. 1.16.16. Transposition of the great arteries: surgery. Mustard procedure: **a** pre-measured metal trousers for the preparation of the Teflon patch to be used as intra-atrial baffle; the leg for the inferior vena cava is larger than the leg for the superior vena cava, **b** Teflon patch (trousers shaped) to be used as intra-atrial baffle, **c** as an alternative, an autologous or heterologous pericardial patch can be used as intra-atrial baffle, **d** after a longitudinal right atriotomy, the atrial septum is completely excised and the roof of the coronary sinus is incised, **e** exposure of the intra-atrial anatomy, to identify pulmonary veins, superior and inferior vena cava and the coronary sinus, **f** the anastomosis of the intra-atrial baffle begins with the suture of the patch to separate the left pulmonary veins from the mitral valve, **g** the anastomosis of the intra-atrial baffle continues with the suture of the patch to separate the mitral valve from the tricuspid valve, **h** the suture of the intra-atrial baffle is now directed to cover the orifice of the superior vena cava, in order to deviate the systemic venous return from the superior vena cava into the mitral valve, **i** the suture of the intra-atrial baffle around the orifice of the superior vena cava is completed, **j** the suture of the intra-atrial baffle is now directed to cover the orifice of the inferior vena cava, in order to also deviate the systemic venous return from the inferior vena cava into the mitral valve, **k** the suture of the intra-atrial baffle around the orifice of the inferior vena cava is now completed; the systemic venous return is now completely deviated into the mitral valve, left ventricle, pulmonary artery. On the side of the intra-atrial baffle the pulmonary veins remain free to drain the pulmonary venous return around the intra-atrial baffle into the tricuspid valve, right ventricle, aorta, **l** the procedure of atrial rerouting is completed by enlargement of the new pulmonary venous atrium with a heterologous pericardial patch, in order to provide an unrestricted channel from the pulmonary veins to the tricuspid valve

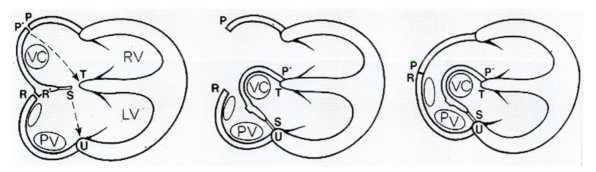

Fig. 1.16.17. Transposition of the great arteries: surgery. Senning procedure: diagram of the principle of atrial rerouting in the Senning procedure, with the line of the right atriotomy (P-P'), the incision on the side of the atrial septum (R-R'), the atrial septum used as a flap, together with the lateral right atrial wall, in a way to rerouting the systemic venous return from the superior and inferior vena cava to the mitral valve, left ventricle, pulmonary artery; the pulmonary venous channel is completed by suturing the anterior edge of the right atrial incision to the lateral edge of the left atrial incision (*LV* left ventricle, *PV* pulmonary veins, *RV* right ventricle, *VC* venae cavae)

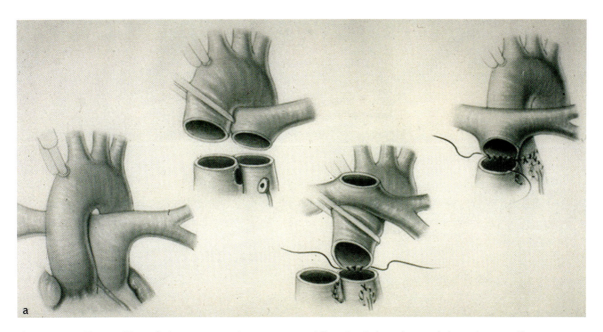

Fig. 1.16.18. Transposition of the great arteries: surgery. Jatene operation (arterial switch): **a** diagram of the arterial switch operation: transection of aorta and pulmonary artery above the sinuses, excision of the coronary arteries from the aortic root with a botton of aorta and implantation in the new aortic root (old pulmonary artery). The pulmonary artery bifurcation is brought anteriorly to the aorta (*Lecompte maneuver*) and the ascending aorta is anastomosed to the new aortic root. A portion of pericardium is utilized to close the defects created in the neo-pulmonary root (old aorta) by the excision of the coronary arteries, and the pulmonary artery bifurcation is anastomosed to the new pulmonary artery root

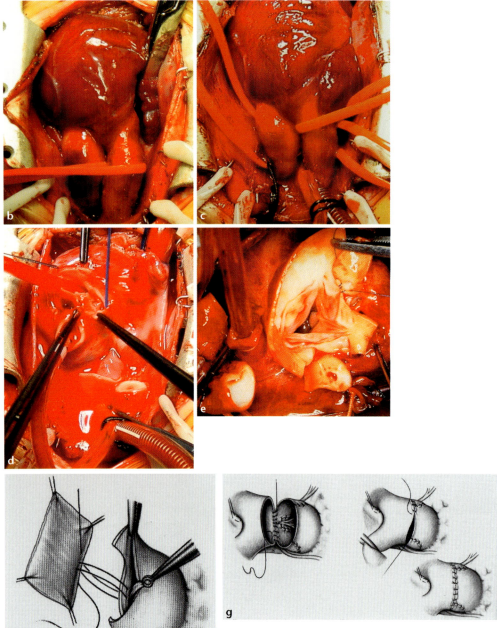

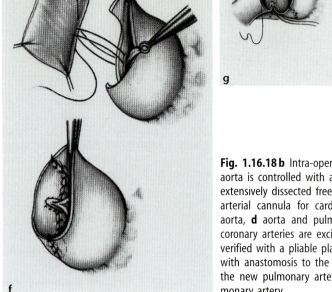

Fig. 1.16.18 b Intra-operative photograph: preparation for arterial switch; the aorta is controlled with a red elastic vessel loop, **c** the pulmonary arteries are extensively dissected free and controlled with red elastic vessel loops, and the arterial cannula for cardiopulmonary bypass is inserted into the ascending aorta, **d** aorta and pulmonary artery are transected above the sinuses, the coronary arteries are excised from the aortic root with a botton of aorta and verified with a pliable plastic probe, **e** implantation of the first coronary artery with anastomosis to the new aortic root, **f** pericardial patch reconstruction of the new pulmonary artery root, **g** completed reconstruction of the new pulmonary artery

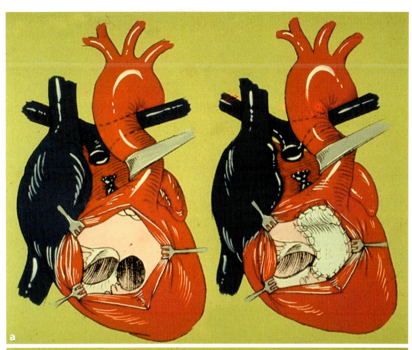

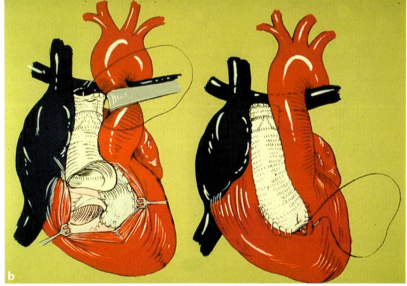

Fig. 1.16.19. Transposition of the great arteries: surgery. Rastelli operation: **a** schematic drawing of the construction of the intracardiac Dacron tunnel connecting the left ventricle to the aorta, **b** the reconstruction of the continuity between the right ventricle and the pulmonary artery with a valved conduit (reproduced with permission from Dr. Carlo Marcelletti)

■ **Rastelli operation** (Figs. 1.16.19 and 1.16.20): After right ventriculotomy, the ventricular septal defect is closed with a prosthetic patch (generally PTFE) by creating a tunnel which connects the left ventricle to the aorta, and continuity between right ventricle and pulmonary artery is obtained with a biological valved conduit.

■ **Lecompte procedure (or REV = Réparation à l'Etage Ventriculaire)** (Fig. 1.16.21): After right ventriculotomy and infundibular resection, the left ventricle is connected to the aorta by closure of ventricular septal defect with a straight patch. After transection and shortening of the ascending aorta and transfer of the pulmonary artery bifurcation anteriorly to the aorta (*Lecompte maneuver*), the right ventricle-to-pulmonary artery continu-

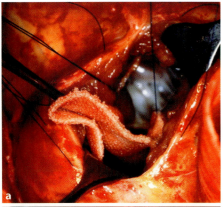

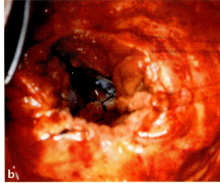

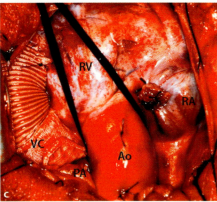

Fig. 1.16.20. Transposition of the great arteries: surgery. Rastelli operation: **a** intra-operative photograph of the construction of the intracardiac Dacron tunnel connecting the left ventricle to the aorta, **b** completion of the intracardiac Dacron tunnel connecting the left ventricle to the aorta, **c** completion of the operation with a valved conduit reconstructing the continuity between the right ventricle and the right pulmonary artery (*Ao* aorta, *PA* pulmonary artery, *RA* right atrium, *RV* right ventricle, *VC* valved conduit)

ity is obtained with reimplantation of the transected pulmonary artery directly on the right ventricle for its posterior wall, while the anterior aspect is connected to the rest of the right ventriculotomy with a monocusp pericardial patch.

■ **Damus-Kaye-Stansel procedure** (Fig. 1.16.22): The pulmonary artery is transected proximal to the bifurcation and end-to-side anastomosed to the ascending aorta, diverting the left ventricular outflow to the systemic circulation; the ventricular septal defect is closed with a prosthetic patch and the continuity between the right ventricle and the pulmonary artery is obtained with a biological valved conduit implanted between the right ventriculotomy and the pulmonary artery bifurcation.

■ Potential complications

■ **Atrioseptectomy:** Supraventricular arrhythmias, inadequate *mixing* at atrial level.

■ **Atrial rerouting:** Arrhythmias: a substantial percentage of patients after 10–15 years have rhythm disturbances: 25% have disorders of the sino-atrial node and 1% per year develop late sudden death; complete atrioventricular block would require a pacemaker implantation.

Tricuspid valve regurgitation: more frequent with ventricular septal defect closure done through the tricuspid valve.

Right (systemic) ventricular dysfunction: this occurs because the morphological right ventricle is functioning as the systemic ventricle, in addition to possible tricuspid valve regurgitation.

Residual or recurrent obstruction of the pulmonary or the systemic venous return may be possible, because of stenosis of the new caval or pulmonary venous channels.

■ **Arterial switch (Jatene operation):** Residual or recurrent coronary arteries stenosis (because of the coronary artery reimplantation),

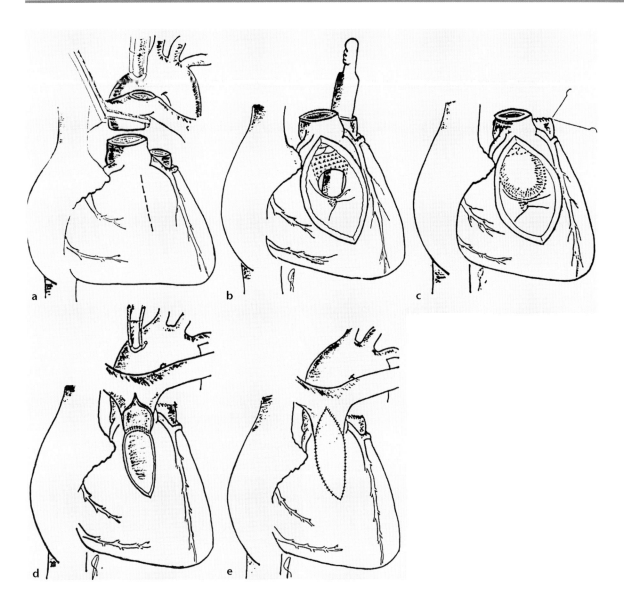

Fig. 1.16.21. Transposition of the great arteries: surgery. Lecompte procedure (or REV = Réparation à l'Etage Ventriculaire): **a** schematic drawing of the transection and shortening of the ascending aorta, the transfer of the pulmonary artery bifurcation anteriorly to the aorta (*Lecompte maneuver*) and the longitudinal right ventriculotomy, **b** through the right ventriculotomy, the infundibular resection is guided by a Hegar dilator introduced into the left ventricle from the transected ascending aorta, **c** after infundibular resection, the left ventricle is connected to the aorta by closure of the ventricular septal defect with a straight patch, **d** the continuity between the right ventricle and the pulmonary artery is obtained with reimplantation of the posterior wall of the transected pulmonary artery directly on the right ventricle, corresponding to the edge of the right ventriculotomy, **e** the continuity between the right ventricle and the pulmonary artery is completed with the connection of the anterior aspect of the pulmonary artery to the rest of the right ventriculotomy with a monocusp pericardial patch

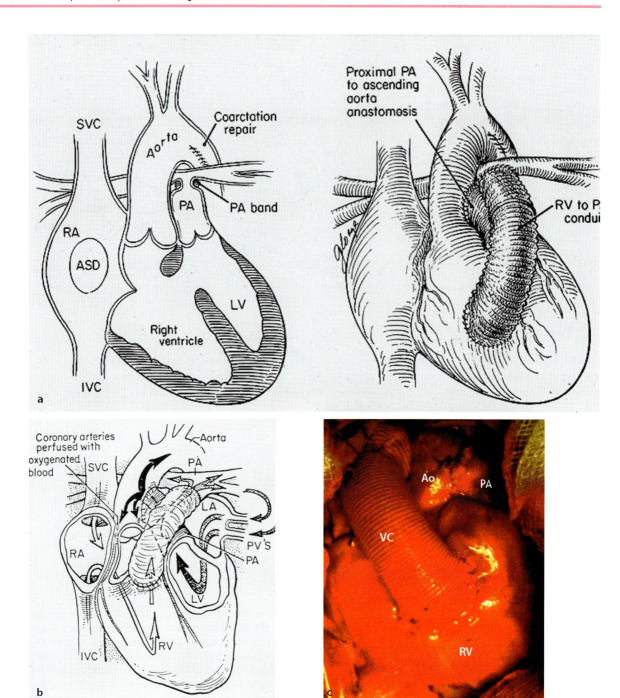

Fig. 1.16.22. Transposition of the great arteries: surgery. Da-mus-Kaye-Stansel procedure: **a** schematic drawing of the pre-operative (A) and the post-operative (B) anatomy, after transection of the main pulmonary artery at the level of the bifurcation and its end-to-side anastomosis to the lateral side of the ascending aorta; after patch closure of the ventricular septal defect, the continuity between the right ventricle and the pulmonary artery is obtained with a valved conduit im-planted between the right ventriculotomy and the pulmo-nary artery bifurcation, **b** shematic drawing of the post-op-erative circulation (*ASD* atrial septal defect, *IVC* inferior vena cava, *LA* left atrium, *LV* left ventricle, *PA* pulmonary artery, *PVs* pulmonary veins, *RA* right atrium, *RV* right ventricle, *SVC* superior vena cava) (photographs courtesy of Dr. Carlo Mar-celletti), **c** intra-operative photograph, with the end-to-side pulmonary artery-to-ascending aorta anastomosis and the right ventricle-to-pulmonary artery valved conduit (*Ao* aorta, *PA* pulmonary artery, *RV* right ventricle, *VC* valved conduit)

residual or recurrent obstruction of the new right ventricular outflow tract (more frequent) or the new left ventricular outflow tract (much more rare).

∎ **Rastelli operation:** Residual or recurrent ventricular septal defect, residual or recurrent obstruction of the new left ventricular outflow tract, obstruction of the right ventricle-to-pulmonary artery valved conduit, complete atrio-ventricular block.

∎ **Lecompte procedure (or REV = Réparation à l'Etage Ventriculaire):** Residual or recurrent ventricular septal defect, residual or recurrent obstruction of the new right ventricle outflow tract, complete atrio-ventricular block.

∎ **Damus-Kaye-Stansel procedure:** Residual or recurrent ventricular septal defect, residual or recurrent obstruction of the new left ventricular outflow tract, late regurgitation of the systemic (aortic or pulmonary) valves, obstruction of the right ventricle-to-pulmonary artery valved conduit, complete atrio-ventricular block.

Neurological abnormalities can be relatively frequent in children with pre-operative prolonged cyanosis or intravenous manipulations, for example, cardiac catheterization which may result in emboli to the central nervous system from the venous circulation. As many as 10–20% of the patients develop a lower IQ and motor development delay.

∎ References

Al Qethamy HO, Aizaz K, Aboelnazar SA, Hijab S, Al Faraidi Y (2002) Two-stage arterial switch operation: is late ever too late? Asian Cardiovasc Thorac Ann 10:235–239

Amodeo A, Corno AF, Marino B, Carta MG, Marcelletti C (1990) Combined repair of transposed great arteries and total anomalous pulmonary venous connection. Ann Thorac Surg 50:820–821

Anderson RH, Tynan M (1984) Complete transposition. The significance of describing separately connexions, arterial relationships and infundibular morphology. Int J Cardiol 5:19–20

Blalock A, Hanlon CR (1950) The surgical treatment of complete transposition of the aorta and the pulmonary artery. Surg Gynecol Obstet 90:1–15

Castaneda AR, Norwood WI, Lang P, Sanders SP (1984) Transposition of the great arteries and intact ventricular septum: anatomic correction in the neonate. Ann Thorac Surg 38:438

Chiu IS, Wang JK, Wu MH (2002) Spiral arterial switch operation in transposition of the great arteries. J Thorac Cardiovasc Surg 124:1050–1052

Corno AF, Picardo S, Ballerini L, Gugliantini P, Marcelletti C (1985) Bronchial compression by dilated pulmonary artery: surgical treatment. J Thorac Cardiovasc Surg 90:706–720

Corno AF, Carotti A, Marino B, Rossi E, Marcelletti C (1987) Left ventricular outflow tract obstruction in patients with transposition of the great arteries with or without ventricular septal defect. Pediat Cardiol (Abstracts) 24

Corno AF, Laks H, George B, Williams RG (1987) Use of in situ pericardium for surgical relief of pulmonary venous obstruction following Mustard's operation. Ann Thorac Surg 43:443–444

Corno AF, Parisi F, Marino B, Ballerini L, Marcelletti C (1987) Palliative Mustard operation: an expanded horizon. Eur J Cardiothorac Surg 1:144–147

Corno AF, Giamberti A, Giannico S, Marino B, Picardo S, Ballerini L, Marcelletti C (1988) Long-term results after extracardiac valved conduits implanted for complex congenital heart disease. J Card Surg 3:495–500

Corno AF, Carta MG, Giannico S (1989) Pulmonary artery banding through median sternotomy. Cl Res 37:91A

Corno AF, George B, Pearl J, Laks H (1989) Surgical options for complex transposition of the great arteries. J Am Coll Cardiol 14:742–749

Corno AF, Giamberti A, Giannico S, Marino B, Rossi E, Marcelletti C, Kirklin JK (1990) Airway obstruction associated with congenital heart disease in infancy. J Thorac Cardiovasc Surg 99:1091–1098

Corno AF (1991) Indications for atrial or arterial switch operation. In: D'Alessandro LC (ed) Heart Surgery 1991. CESI, Rome, Italy, pp 229–336

Corno AF, Papa M, Santoro F, Zoia E (1993) Aneurysm of the membranous ventricular septum in transposition of the great arteries. J Thorac Cardiovasc Surg 105:369–371

Corno AF, Da Cruz E, Lal AB, Milella L, Wilson N (1998) Controlled reoxygenation for cyanotic patients. In: Imai Y, Momma K (eds) Proceedings of 2nd World Congress of PCCS. Futura Publishing Co., Armonk, NY, pp 1127–1129

Corno AF, Hurni M, Payot M, von Segesser LK (1999) Modified Blalock-Taussig shunt with compensatory properties. Ann Thorac Surg 67:269–270

Corno AF, von Segesser LK (1999) Is hypothermia necessary in pediatric cardiac surgery? Eur J Cardiothorac Surg 15:110–111

Corno AF, von Segesser LK (2001) Transposition of great arteries and single coronary artery: a new surgical technique for the arterial switch operation. Swiss Med Wkly 131:47–49

Corno AF (2001) Lecompte procedure. Ann Thorac Surg 72:180–181 (invited commentary)

Corno AF, Hurni M, Griffin H, Galal OM, Payot M, Sekarski N, Tozzi P, von Segesser LK (2002) Bovine jugular vein as right ventricle-to-pulmonary artery valved conduit. J Heart Valve Dis 11:242–247

Corno AF, Hurni M, Payot M, Sekarski N, Tozzi P, von Segesser LK (2003) Adequate left ventricular preparation allows for arterial switch despite late referral. Cardiol Young 13:49

Crupi GC, Anderson RH, Ho YS, Lincoln C (1979) Complete transposition of the great arteries with intact ventricular septum and left ventricular outflow tract obstruction. Surgical management and anatomic considerations. J Thorac Cardiovasc Surg 78:730–738

Damus PS (1975) Letter to the Editor. Ann Thorac Surg 20:724–725

Di Carlo DC, di Donato RM, Corno AF, Ballerini L, Marcelletti C (1987) The Damus-Kaye-Stansel procedure in infancy. Pediat Cardiol (Abstracts) 10

Ferencz C, Rubin JD, McCarter RJ (1985) Congenital heart disease: prevalence at livebirth. The Baltimore-Washington infant study. Am J Epidemiol 121:31–36

Fyler DC, Buckley LP, Hellenbrand WE, Cohn HE (1980) Report of the New England Regional Infant Care Program. Pediatrics 65(Suppl):375–461

Gittenberger-de Groot AC, Sauer U, Oppenheimer-Dekker A, Quaegebeur J (1983) Coronary arterial anatomy in transposition of the great arteries: a morphological study. Pediatr Cardiol 4(Suppl):15–24

Hoffman JIE, Kaplan S (2002) The incidence of congenital heart disease. J Am Coll Cardiol 39:1890–1900

Horisberger J, Jegger D, Boone Y, Seigneul I, Pierrel N, Hurni M, Corno AF, von Segesser LK (1999) Impact of a remote pump head on neonatal priming volumes. Perfusion 14:351–356

Hovels-Gurich HH, Vasquez-Jimenez JF, Silvestri A, Schumacher K, Minkenberg R, Duchateau J, Messmer BJ, von Bernuth G, Seghaye MC (2002) Production of proinflammatory cytokines and myocardial dysfunction after arterial switch operation in neonates with transposition of the great arteries. J Thorac Cardiovasc Surg 124:811–820

Hutter PA, Kreb DL, Mantel SF, Hitchcock JF, Meijboom EJ, Bennink GB (2002) Twenty-five years' experience with the arterial switch operation. J Thorac Cardiovasc Surg 124:790–797

Jatene AD, Fontes VF, Paulista PP, Souza LCB, Neger F, Galantier M, Sousa JE (1976) Anatomic correction of transposition of the great vessels. J Thorac Cardiovasc Surg 72:364–370

Jonas RA, Giglia TM, Sanders SP, Wernovsky G, Nadal-Ginard B, Mayer JE, Castaneda AR (1980) Rapid, two-stage arterial switch for transposition of the great arteries and intact ventricular septum beyond the neonatal period. Circulation 80(Suppl I):203

Kaye MP (1975) Anatomic correction of transposition of the great arteries. Mayo Clin Proc 50:638–640

Lecompte Y, Neveux JY, Leca F, Zannini L, Tu TV, Duboys Y, Jarreau MM (1982) Reconstruction of the pulmonary outflow tract without prosthetic conduit. J Thorac Cardiovasc Surg 84:727

Lecompte Y, Zannini L, Hazan E, Jarreau MM, Bex JP, Tu TV, Neveux JY (1981) Anatomic correction of transposition of the great arteries. J Thorac Cardiovasc Surg 82:629

Lecompte Y, Bex JP (1985) Repair of transposition of the great arteries with ventricular septal defect and left ventricular outflow tract obstruction. J Thorac Cardiovasc Surg 90:151–154

Lecompte Y (2002) Rastelli repair for transposition of the great arteries: still the best choice? J Thorac Cardiovasc Surg 123:211–223

Lindesmith GG, Stiles QR, Tucker BL, Gallagher ME, Stanton RE, Meyer BW (1972) The Mustard operation as a palliative procedure. J Thorac Cardiovasc Surg 63:75

Mair DD, Ritter DG (1973) Factors influencing systemic arterial oxygen saturation in complete transposition of the great arteries. Am J Cardiol 31:742–748

Mair DD, Ritter DG, Danielson GK, Wallace RB, McGoon DC (1976) The palliative Mustard operation: rationale and results. Am J Cardiol 37:762

Marcelletti C, Corno F, Losekoot TG, Olthof H, Schuller J, Bulterijs AHK, Becker AE (1980) Condotti extracardiaci: indicazioni, tecniche e risultati immediati. G Ital Cardiol 10:1041–1054

Marcelletti C, Corno AF (1981) Extracardiac conduits: indications, techniques and early results. 33th Herhalings Cursus Kindergeneeskunde, Amsterdam(Abstracts)

Marino B, Corno AF, Carotti A, Pasquini L, Giannico S, Guccione P, Bevilacqua M, De Simone G, Marcelletti C (1990) Pediatric cardiac surgery guided by echocardiography. Scand J Thorac Cardiovasc Surg 24:197–201

Marino B, Capolino R, Digilio MC, Di Donato R (2002) Transposition of the great arteries in asplenia and polysplenia phenotypes. Am J Med Genet 110:292–294

Massoudy P, Baltalarli A, de Leval MR, Cook A, Neudorf U, Derrick G, McCarthy KP, Anderson RH (2002) Anatomic variability in coronary arterial distribution with regard to the arterial switch procedure. Circulation 106:1980–1984

Mustard WT, Chute AL, Keith JD, Sivek A, Rowe RD, Vlad P (1954) A surgical approach to transposition of the great vessels with extracorporeal circuit. Surgery 36:39–51

Nikaidoh H (1984) Aortic translocation and biventricular outflow tract reconstruction. A new surgical repair for transposition of the great arteries associated with ventricular septal defect and pulmonary stenosis. J Thorac Cardiovasc Surg 88: 365

Oskarsson G, Pesonen E, Munkhammar P, Sandstrom S, Jogi P (2002) Normal coronary flow reserve after arterial switch operation for transposition of the great arteries: an intracoronary Doppler guidewire study. Circulation 106:1696–1702

Pasquali SK, Hasselblad V, Li JS, Kong DF, Sanders SP (2002) Coronary artery pattern and outcome of arterial switch operation for transposition of the great arteries: a meta-analysis. Circulation 106:2575–2580

Rashkind WJ, Miller WW (1966) Creation of an atrial septal defect without thoracotomy: a palliative approach to complete transposition of the great arteries. JAMA 196:991–992

Rastelli GC (1969) A new approach to anatomic repair of transposition of the great arteries. Mayo Clin Proc 44:1

Sakata R, Lecompte Y, Batisse A, Borromée L, Durandy Y (1988) Anatomic repair of anomalies of ventriculo-arterial connection associated with ventricular septal defect. J Thorac Cardiovasc Surg 95:90–95

Senning A (1959) Surgical correction of transposition of the great vessels. Surgery 45:966–980

Stansel HC (1975) A new operation for d-loop transposition of the great vessels. Ann Thorac Surg 19:565–567

Stark J, de Leval MR, Taylor JF (1976) Mustard operation and creation of ventricular septal defect in two patients with transposition of the great arteries, intact ventricular septum and pulmonary vascular disease. Am J Cardiol 38:524

Yacoub MH, Radley-Smith R (1978) Anatomy of the coronary arteries in transposition of the great arteries and methods for their transfer in anatomical correction. Thorax 33:418–424

Yacoub MH, Radley-Smith R, Maclaurin R (1977) Two-stage operation for anatomical correction of transposition of the great arteries with intact ventricular septum. Lancet 1:1275

Incidence

Hypoplastic left heart syndrome is the 8th most common congenital heart disease. It occurs in 0.16–0.68/1000 live births (4% of all congenital heart diseases at all ages).

Morphology

The morphological features (Fig. 1.17.1) of the hypoplastic left heart syndrome are the following:
▌ Mitral atresia or severe stenosis
▌ Aortic atresia or severe stenosis
▌ Left ventricular hypoplasia or aplasia
▌ Left atrial hypoplasia
▌ Restrictive interatrial communication
▌ Patent ductus arteriosus
▌ Aortic coarctation
▌ Right atrial dilatation
▌ Right ventricular dilatation and hypertrophy

The apex is formed by the right ventricle and the epicardial course of the left anterior descending coronary artery defines a very small or non-existent left ventricle.

The ascending aorta may be as small as 1 or 2 mm, but large enough to supply blood to the coronary arteries in a retrograde fashion.

A patent foramen ovale is generally small, with herniation of the valve of the septum primum from left-to-right, or even closed. Premature closure of the patent foramen ovale is usually accompanied by severe hypoplasia of the left heart cavities. Endocar-dial fibroelastosis may also be present. Left ventricle to coronary arteries connections have been described.

The ductus arteriosus is widely patent, serving as a downward-directed conduit from the main pulmonary artery to the descending thoracic aorta.

The neonates are generally not born with aortic coarctation, but it frequently develops (80% of cases). Obstructions at the level of the aortic arch are frequently present.

Associated anomalies

Dextrocardia and isomerism are uncommon, as well as juxtaposition of the auricular appendages. Rare is the incidence of associated partial anomalous pulmonary venous connection. Aortic arch interruption is very rare.

Possible is the association with dominant right form of atrio-ventricular septal defect, double outlet right ventricle or aortic-left ventricular tunnel.

Morphological anomalies of the tricuspid valve are unusual, despite the frequent presence of tricuspid valve regurgitation. Extremely rare is the association with pulmonary valve stenosis. Extremely rare is the presence of a ventricular septal defect.

Pathophysiology

Survival in these patients depends on the patency of the ductus arteriosus and on an adequate interatrial communication.

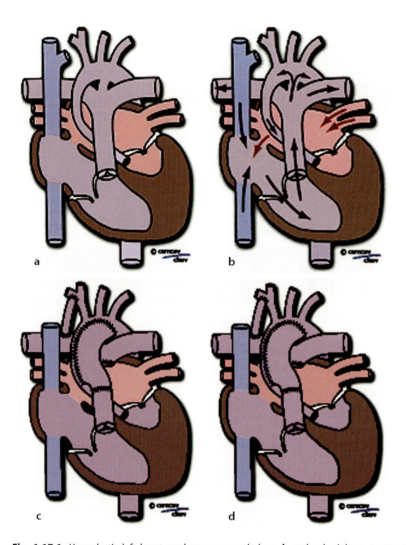

Fig. 1.17.1. Hypoplastic left heart syndrome: **a** morphology, **b** pathophysiology, **c** surgery, Norwood procedure, **d** Sano variation

The right ventricle provides blood flow to the pulmonary arteries and to the systemic circulation through the patent ductus arteriosus. The systemic distal circulation is generally well perfused through the patent ductus arteriosus. The proximal systemic circulation is perfused through the patent ductus arteriosus in a retrograde fashion, frequently with obstructions at the level of the aortic isthmus and/or the aortic arch. The coronary arteries receive retrograde perfusion through the hypoplastic ascending aorta.

The pulmonary blood flow depends upon the pulmonary vascular resistance which in turn depends upon the size of the patent fora-

men ovale. When the patent foramen ovale is restrictive, the left atrial pressure remains elevated, causing increased pulmonary vascular resistance. Only increased pulmonary vascular resistance can allow maintenance of adequate systemic perfusion through the patent foramen ovale.

∎ Diagnosis

∎ **Clinical pattern:** without the administration of prostaglandin to maintain patency of the ductus arteriosus, these neonates can present in a condition of poor cardiac output shortly after birth, with progressive me-

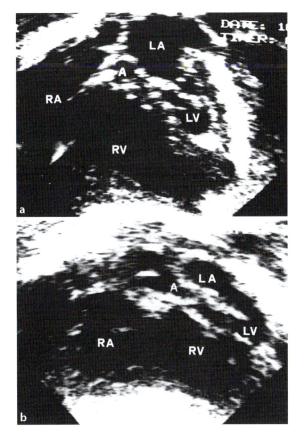

Fig. 1.17.2. Hypoplastic left heart syndrome: echocardiography. **a** long-axis view showing the extreme hypoplasia of the left ventricle and ascending aorta and the dilatation of right ventricle and right atrium, **b** long-axis sub-xiphoid view showing the extreme hypoplasia of the left ventricle and ascending aorta and the dilatation of right ventricle and right atrium (*A* aorta, *LA* left atrium, *LV* left ventricle, *RA* right atrium, *RV* right ventricle) (reproduced with permission from Marino B, Thiene G (1990) Atlante di anatomia ecocardiografica delle cardiopatie congenite, USES, Firenze)

tabolic acidosis, poor renal perfusion and an increase in intravenous volume, hyperkalemia; hyperkalemia associated with hypoglycemia and decreased coronary blood flow due to the constriction of the patent ductus arteriosus can lead to severe myocardial injury and death; neonates with more stable patent ductus arteriosus present with dyspnea, tachypnea, pallor or cyanosis, cool skin, nasal flaring, subcostal and intercostal retractions, basal rales at ventilation; very poor central and peripheral pulses and extreme hepatomegaly are common; the second heart sound is accentuated and single.

▪ **Electrocardiogram:** right axis deviation, conspicuous right ventricular hypertrophy.

▪ **Chest X-ray:** moderate cardiomegaly; increased pulmonary blood flow and congestion or edema.

▪ **Echocardiogram:** long-axis sub-xiphoid view shows the extreme hypoplasia of the left ventricle and ascending aorta and the dilatation of right ventricle and right atrium (Fig. 1.17.2); when a Norwood operation is considered, the following aspects need to be evaluated:
– presence and degree of tricuspid valve regurgitation
– presence of aortic coarctation and/or transverse aortic arch hypoplasia
– pulmonary valve stenosis
– pulmonary venous obstruction
– right ventricular function.

▪ **Cardiac catheterization:** needed to perform an angiography to visualize ascending aorta and aortic arch (Fig. 1.17.3).

▪ Indications for surgical treatment

Since these neonates typically present with acidosis and shock, they need tracheal intubation and mechanical ventilation, with correction of acidosis and prostaglandin infusion to increase the pulmonary blood flow and maintain the patency of the ductus arteriosus.

As the ductus arteriosus is opened by prostaglandin, the pulmonary blood flow increases significantly, therefore the pulmonary vasodilatation provided by the prostaglandin needs to be controlled by increasing the pulmonary vascular resistance. This could be obtained by hypercarbia, controlled acidosis and mild hypoxia. Hypercarbia can be achieved by providing subambient oxygen through mixing carbon dioxide or nitrogen with room air.

Surgical management includes different options:

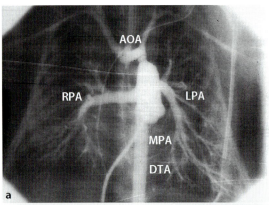

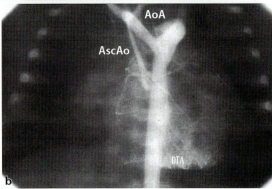

Fig. 1.17.3. Hypoplastic left heart syndrome: angiography. **a** antero-posterior view with injection in the main pulmonary artery showing opacification of the branches of the pulmonary artery and, with perfusion through the patent ductus arteriosus, opacification of the descending thoracic aorta and retrograde perfusion of the aortic isthmus, with aortic coarctation, of the aortic arch with the neck vessel and of the very hypoplastic ascending aorta, **b** antero-posterior view with injection through the main pulmonary artery and patent ductus arteriosus showing the descending thoracic aorta, retrograde perfusion of the aortic isthmus, of the aortic arch with the neck vessel and of the very hypoplastic ascending aorta with the coronary arteries (*AoA* aortic arch, *AscAo* ascending aorta, *DTA* descending thoracic aorta, *LPA* left pulmonary artery, *MPA* main pulmonary artery, *RPA* right pulmonary artery)

■ Palliation: *stent of the ductus arteriosus and bilateral pulmonary artery banding.*

■ Univentricular type of repair in three stages: the first stage is the *Norwood procedure,* followed by a bi-directional Glenn (end-to-side anastomosis of the superior vena cava to the right pulmonary artery) and then by a modified Fontan procedure (total cavo-pulmonary connection by extra-cardiac or intra-cardiac connection of the inferior vena cava to the pulmonary artery).

■ Heart transplantation.

■ **Stent of the ductus arteriosus and bilateral pulmonary artery banding:** This palliative approach, consisting of stenting the ductus arteriosus to maintain the patency and surgical (or intravascular) bilateral pulmonary artery banding to maintain adequate systemic perfusion through the ductus arteriosus, has been recently proposed with two potential targets: a) to improve the clinical condition of the neonate, particularly when very critical with signs of multi-organ failure, to increase the chances of tolerating a subsequent Norwood type of procedure; b) to allow stabilization for a period long enough that a donor heart becomes available for heart transplantation.

■ **Norwood procedure:** The Norwood procedure consists of an initial palliative procedure (first stage) in view of a univentricular type repair. Palliation includes using the pulmonary valve and proximal main pulmonary artery as neo-aorta, by transecting the distal main pulmonary artery and connecting the proximal main pulmonary artery to the aortic arch and ascending aorta. Then the pulmonary blood flow is provided by a systemic to pulmonary artery shunt from the right subclavian artery or the innominate artery to the right pulmonary artery. In addition, the atrial septum is removed surgically to create an unrestricted interatrial communication and the patent ductus arteriosus is divided. Even in the absence of evident aortic coarctation, the area of aortic isthmus can be bypassed by an aortic homograft, to avoid the risk of recurrent aortic coarctation.

■ **Heart transplantation:** Heart transplantation in hypoplastic left heart syndrome is not different from routine heart transplantation, with two exceptions: a) the need for a special technique for cardiopulmonary by-

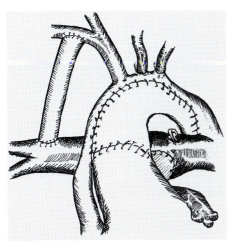

Fig. 1.17.4. Hypoplastic left heart syndrome: surgery. Norwood procedure, first stage

pass, due to the presence of ductal dependency of the systemic perfusion; b) the need for reconstruction of the aortic arch and aortic isthmus.

▪ Surgical treatment (on cardiopulmonary bypass)

▪ **Norwood procedure** (Fig. 1.17.4): Despite recent proposals for avoiding deep hypothermia and circulatory arrest, the original surgical technique includes a period of deep hypothermia and circulatory arrest. After removal of the single venous cannula, through the same incision of the right atrium used for the cannula, the atrial septum is excised (atrioseptectomy). On circulatory arrest the patent ductus arteriosus is divided, and the corresponding opening remaining on the aortic isthmus is longitudinally incised, distally across the area of the isthmus and proximally to widely open the aortic arch and ascending aorta. The main pulmonary artery is divided in correspondence of the bifurcation, and the remaining opening on the bifurcation is closed with a biological

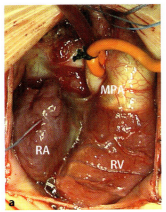
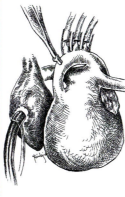
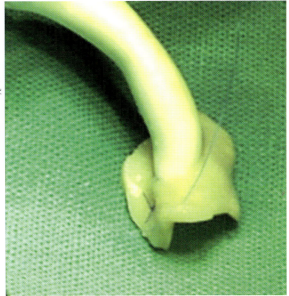
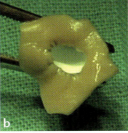
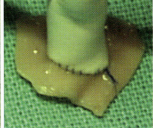

Fig. 1.17.5. Hypoplastic left heart syndrome: surgery. Norwood procedure, first stage, with the Sano variation. **a** aortic cannulation, feasible only when allowed by the size of the ascending aorta, instead of the conventional cannulation of the main pulmonary artery, with systemic perfusion through the patent ductus arteriosus (*MPA* main pulmonary artery, *RA* right atrium, *RV* right ventricle), **b** preparation of the distal end of the PTFE prosthesis with a button of biological tissue (homograft or pericardium) to be anastomosed to the pulmonary artery bifurcation

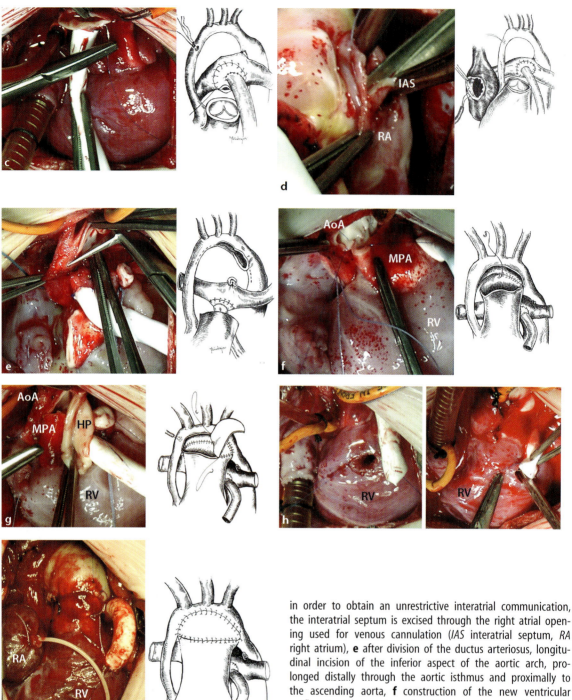

Fig. 1.17.5. **c** after closure of the ductus arteriosus and division of the main pulmonary artery in correspondence of the bifurcation, anastomosis of the distal end of the PTFE prosthesis with a button of biological tissue (homograft or pericardium) to the pulmonary artery bifurcation, **d** atrioseptectomy: in order to obtain an unrestrictive interatrial communication, the interatrial septum is excised through the right atrial opening used for venous cannulation (*IAS* interatrial septum, *RA* right atrium), **e** after division of the ductus arteriosus, longitudinal incision of the inferior aspect of the aortic arch, prolonged distally through the aortic isthmus and proximally to the ascending aorta, **f** construction of the new ventricular outflow tract by anastomosis of the posterior wall of the main pulmonary artery to the posterior wall of the incised aortic arch (*AoA* aortic arch, *MPA* main pulmonary artery, *RV* right ventricle), **g** completion of the new ventricular outflow tract by joining the anterior wall of the main pulmonary artery to the anterior wall of the aortic arch by interposition of a patch of homograft (*HP* homograft patch), **h** proximal anastomosis of the PTFE tubular prosthesis to the opening on the anterior wall of the right ventricle, **i** final appearance after decannulation (photographs courtesy of Dr. Edward Malec)

patch (pericardium or homograft). The neo-aorta is constructed by connecting the proximal main pulmonary artery to the aortic arch and ascending aorta, either directly or with a longitudinally opened aortic homograft, to entirely bypass the area of the aortic isthmus. After restoring the cardiopulmonary bypass and during rewarming, the pulmonary blood flow is provided by a systemic to pulmonary artery shunt from the right subclavian artery or the innominate artery to the right pulmonary artery (modified Blalock-Taussig shunt).

Within the last few years, alternative techniques have been proposed with cerebral perfusion through a PTFE tubular prosthesis end-to-side anastomosed to the innominate artery, in order to avoid complete circulatory arrest.

■ **Norwood procedure with the Sano variation** (Fig. 1.17.5): The modified Norwood operation, proposed by Sano and nowadays widely adopted, including Norwood himself, replaces the modified Blalock-Taussig shunt with a tubular prosthesis implanted between the anterior aspect of the right ventricle and the pulmonary artery bifurcation. The advantage is to avoid stealing blood from the coronary arteries during diastole, a complication difficult to manage after the classical Norwood procedure.

Potential complications

■ **Norwood procedure:** The immediate postoperative period is complicated by the very difficult balance between the systemic and pulmonary circulation, in parallel with a single ventricle physiology. Tricuspid regurgitation may develop and become progressive, and this represents a major issue since the right ventricle is functioning as the systemic ventricle. Recurrent aortic coarctation is possible in the case of incomplete resection of residual ductal tissue. Rarely the pulmonary veins may develop progressive stenosis, and the etiology is unclear.

■ **Norwood procedure with the Sano variation:** The main problem reported after this modified technique consists in hypoxia, more evident than after the classic Norwood procedure. Concern remains for the long-term effects on the ventricular function, because of the need for a ventriculotomy on the systemic ventricle.

References

Aiello VD, Ho SY, Anderson RH, Thiene G (1990) Morphologic features of the hypoplastic left heart syndrome: a reappraisal. Pediatr Pathol 10:931

Akintuerk H, Michel-Behnke I, Valeske K, Mueller M, Thul J, Bauer J, Hagel KJ, Kreuder J, Vogt P, Schranz D (2002) Stenting of the arterial duct and banding of the pulmonary arteries: basis for combined Norwood stage I and II repair in hypoplastic left heart. Circulation 105:1099–1103

Azakie T, Merklinger SL, McCrindle BW, van Arsdell GS, Lee KJ, Benson LN, Coles JG, Williams WG (2001) Evolving strategies and improving outcomes of the modified Norwood procedure: a 10-year single-institution experience. Ann Thorac Surg 72:1349–1353

Bailey LL, Nehlsen-Cannarella SL, Conception W, Jolley WB (1985) Baboon-to-human cardiac xenotransplantation in a neonate. JAMA 254:3321–3329

Bailey LL, Nehlsen-Cannarella SL, Doroshow RW, Jacobson JG, Martin RD, Allard MW, Hyde MR, Dang Bui RH, Petry EL (1986) Cardiac allotransplantation in newborn as therapy for hypoplastic left heart syndrome. N Engl J Med 315:949–951

Barnea O, Austin EH, Richman B, Santamore WP (1994) Balancing the circulation: theoretic optimisation of pulmonary/systemic flow ratio in hypoplastic left heart syndrome. J Am Coll Cardiol 24:1376–1381

Bartram U, Grunenfelder J, Van Praagh R (1997) Causes of death after the modified Norwood procedure: a study of 122 postmortem cases. Ann Thorac Surg 64:1795–1802

Bradley SM, Simsic JM, Atz AM (2001) Hemodynamic effects of inspired carbon dioxide after the Norwood procedure. Ann Thorac Surg 72:2088–2094

Chang RK, Chen AY, Klitzner TS (2002) Clinical management of infants with hypoplastic left heart syndrome in the United States, 1988–1997. Pediatrics 110:292–298

Corno AF, Mazzera E, Marino B, Picardo S, Marcelletti C (1989) Bidirectional cavopulmonary anastomosis. J Am Coll Cardiol 13:74A

Corno AF (2000) Surgery for congenital heart disease. Curr Opinion Cardiol 15:238–243

Daebritz SH, Tiete AR, Rassoulian D, Roemer U, Kozlik-Feldmann R, Sachweh J, Netz H, Reichart B (2002) Borderline hypoplastic left heart malformations: Norwood palliation or two-ventricle repair? Thorac Cardiovasc Surg 50:266–270

Ferencz C, Rubin JD, McCarter RJ (1985) Congenital heart disease: prevalence at livebirth. The Baltimore-Washington infant study. Am J Epidemiol 121:31–36

Fyler DC, Buckley LP, Hellenbrand WE, Cohn HE (1980) Report of the New England Regional Infant Care Program. Pediatrics 65(Suppl):375–461

Forbess JM, Cook N, Roth SJ, Mayer JE, Jonas RA (1995) Ten-year institutional experience with palliative surgery for hypoplastic left heart syndrome. Risk factors related to stage I mortality. Circulation 92:II-262–266

Fortuna RS, Chinnock RE, Bailey LL (1999) Heart transplantation among 233 infants during the first six months of life: the Loma Linda experience. Clin Transpl 263

Gaynor JW, Mahle WT, Cohen MI, Ittenbach RF, DeCampli WM, Steven JM, Nicolson SC, Spray TL (2002) Risk factors for mortality after the Norwood procedure. Eur J Cardiothorac Surg 22:82–89

Giannico S, Corno AF, Marino B, Cicini MP, Gagliardi MG, Amodeo A, Picardo S, Marcelletti C (1992) Total extracardiac right heart bypass. Circulation 86(Suppl 2):110–117

Gibbs JL, Wren C, Watterston KG, Hunter S, Hamilton JR (1993) Stenting of the arterial duct combined with banding of the pulmonary arteries and atrial septectomy or septostomy: a new approach to palliation for the hypoplastic left heart syndrome. Br Heart J 69:551–555

Grabitz RG, Joffres MR, Collins-Nakai RL (1988) Congenital heart disease: incidence in the first year of life. The Alberta heritage pediatric cardiology program. Am J Epidemiol 128:381–388

Graziano JN, Heidelberger KP, Ensing GJ, Gomez CA, Ludomirsky A (2002) The influence of a restrictive atrial septal defect on pulmonary vascular morphology in patients with hypoplastic left heart syndrome. Pediatr Cardiol 23:146–151

Gutgesell HP, Gibson J (2002) Management of hypoplastic left heart syndrome in the 1990s. Am J Cardiol 89:842–846

Gutgesell HP (2002) What if it were your child? Am J Cardiol 89:856

Ikle L, Hale K, Fashaw L, Boucek M, Rosenberg AA (2003) Developmental outcome of patients with hypoplastic left heart syndrome treated with heart transplantation. J Pediatr 142:20–25

Imoto Y, Kado H, Shiokawa Y, Minami K, Yasui H (2001) Experience with the Norwood procedure without circulatory arrest. J Thorac Cardiovasc Surg 122:879–882

Ishizaka T, Ohye RG, Suzuki T, Devaney EJ, Bove EL (2003) Bilateral pulmonary artery banding for resuscitation in hypoplastic left heart syndrome. Ann Thorac Surg 75:277–279

Jacobs ML, Blackstone EH, Bailey LL (1998) Intermediate survival in neonates with aortic atresia: a multi-institutional study. The Congenital Heart Surgeons Society. J Thorac Cardiovasc Surg 116:417–431

Jenkins PC, Flanagan MF, Jenkins KJ, Sargent JD, Canter CE, Chinnock RE, Vincent RN, Tosteson AN, O'Connor GT (2000) Survival analysis and risk factors for mortality in transplantation and staged surgery for hypoplastic left heart syndrome. J Am Coll Cardiol 36:1178–1185

Jonas RA, Lang P, Hansen DD, Hickey P, Castaneda AR (1986) First-stage palliation of hypoplastic left heart syndrome: the importance of coarctation and shunt size. J Thorac Cardiovasc Surg 92:6–13

Kishimoto H, Kawahira Y, Kawata H, Miura T, Iwai S, Mori T (1999) The modified Norwood palliation on a beating heart. J Thorac Cardiovasc Surg 118:1130–1132

Korkola SJ, Tchervenkov CI, Shum-Tim D (2002) Aortic arch reconstruction without circulatory arrest: review of techniques, applications, and indications. Semin Thorac Cardiovasc Surg Pediatr Card Surg Ann 5:116–125

Lev M, Arcilla R, Rimoldi HJA, Licata RH, Gasul BM (1963) Premature narrowing or closure of the foramen ovale. Am Heart J 65:638–647

Lim C, Kim WH, Kim SC, Rhyu JW, Baek MJ, Oh SS, Ny CY, Kim CW (2003) Aortic arch reconstruction using regional perfusion without circulatory arrest. Eur J Cardiothorac Surg 23:149–155

Mahle WT, Clancy RR, Moss EM, Gerdes M, Jobes DR, Wernovsky G (2000) Neurodevelopmental outcome and lifestyle assessment in school-aged and adolescent children with hypoplastic left heart syndrome. Pediatrics 105:1082–1089

Marcelletti C, Anderson RH, Becker AE, Corno AF, di Carlo DC, Mazzera E (1986) Pediatric Cardiology, Vol 6. Churchill & Livingstone, London

Marcelletti C, Corno AF, Giannico S, Marino B (1990) Inferior vena cava to pulmonary artery extracardiac conduit: a new form of right heart bypass. J Thorac Cardiovasc Surg 100:228–232

Mazzera E, Corno AF, Picardo S, Di Donato RM, Marino B, Costa D, Marcelletti C (1989) Bidirectional cavopulmonary shunts: clinical applications as staged or definitive palliation. Ann Thorac Surg 47:415–420

Migliavacca F, Pennati G, Dubini G, Fumero R, Pietrabissa R, Urcelay G, Bove EL, Hsia TY, de Leval MR (2001) Modeling of the Norwood circulation: effects of shunt size, vascular resistance, and heart rate. Am J Physiol Heart Circ Physiol 280: H-2076–2086

Milo S, Ho SY, Anderson RH (1980) Hypoplastic left heart syndrome: can this malformation be treated surgically? Thorax 35:351–354

Mitchell MB, Campbell DN, Bielefeld MR, Doremus T (2000) Utility of extracorporeal membrane oxygenation for early graft failure following heart transplantation in infancy. J Heart Lung Transplant 19:934–939

Noona JA, Nadas AS (1958) The hypoplastic left heart syndrome: an analysis of 101 cases. Pediatr Clin North Am 5:1029

Norwood WI, Lang P, Castaneda AR, Campbell DN (1981) Experience with operations for hypoplastic left heart syndrome. J Thorac Cardiovasc Surg 82:511–519

Norwood WI, Lang P, Hansen DD (1983) Physiologic repair of aortic atresia-hypoplastic left heart syndrome. N Engl J Med 308:23–26

Pigula FA (2002) Arch reconstruction without circulatory arrest: scientific basis for continued use and application to patients with arch anomalies. Semin Thorac Cardiovasc Surg Pediatr Card Surg Ann 5:104–115

Pizarro C, Norwood WI (2003) Pulmonary artery banding before Norwood procedure. Ann Thorac Surg 75:1008–1010

Pizarro C, Davis DA, Galantowicz ME, Munro H, Gidding SS, Norwood WI (2002) Stage I palliation for hypoplastic left heart syndrome in low birth weight neonates: can we justify it? Eur J Cardiothorac Surg 21:716–720

Poirier NC, Drummond-Webb JJ, Hisamochi K, Imamura M, Harrison AM, Mee RBB (2000) Modified Norwood procedure with a high-flow cardiopulmonary bypass strategy results in low mortality without late arch obstruction. J Thorac Cardiovasc Surg 120:875–884

Rychik J, Bush DM, Spray TL, Gaynor JW, Wernovsky G (2000) Assessment of pulmonary systemic blood flow ratio after first stage palliation for hypoplastic left heart syndrome: development of a new index with the use of Doppler echocardiography. J Thorac Cardiovasc Surg 120:81–87

Ruiz CE, Gamra H, Zhang HP, Garcia EJ, Boucek MM (1993) Brief report: stenting of the ductus arteriosus as a bridge to cardiac transplantation in infants with the hypoplastic left heart syndrome. N Engl J Med 328:1605–1608

Sade RM, Crawford FA, Fyfe DA (1986) Letter to the editor: symposium on the hypoplastic left heart syndrome. J Thorac Cardiovasc Surg 91:937–939

Sano S, Ishino K, Kawada M, Fujisawa E, Kasahara S, Nakanishi K, Arai S, Hisamochi K, Kamada M, Ohtsuki S (2001) The modified Norwood operation for hypoplastic left heart syndrome using right ventricle-to-pulmonary artery shunt. Cardiol Young 11(Suppl I):21

Starnes VA, Griffin ML, Pitlick PT, Bernstein D, Baum D, Ivens K, Shumway NE (1992) Current approach to hypoplastic left heart syndrome: palliation, transplantation, or both? J Thorac Cardiovasc Surg 104:189–194

Tchervenkov CI, Korkola SJ, Shum-Tim D, Calaritis C, Laliberte E, Reyes TU, Lavoie J (2001) Neonatal aortic arch reconstruction avoiding circulatory arrest and direct arch vessel cannulation. Ann Thorac Surg 72:1615–1620

Tweddell JS, Hoffman GM, Mussatto KA, Fedderly RT, Berger S, Jaquiss RD, Ghanayem NS, Frisbee SJ, Litwin SB (2002) Improved survival of patients undergoing palliation of hypoplastic left heart syndrome: lessons learned from 115 consecutive patients. Circulation 106(Suppl I):182–189

Zeigler VL (2003) Ethical principles and parental choice: treatment options for neonates with hypoplastic left heart syndrome. Pediatr Nurs 29: 65–69

Subject index

Subject index

Antonio F. Corno

Congenital Heart Defects

Decision Making for Surgery

A unique book for all the people taking care of children with congenital heart defects.

- over 500 didactic, clear illustrations visualize the anatomy and key operative steps

- each chapter devoted to a single malformation with incidence, morphology, associated anomalies, pathophysiology, diagnosis, indication on details for surgical treatment, potential complications

- easy-to-follow surgical procedures

- easy-to-read, practical, and uniform style of chapters following 1-defect-is-1-chapter-scheme

- covering all aspects relevant for deciding on treatment

- of great interest to cardiac surgeons, cardiologists, pediatricians and pathologists

- latest essential facts

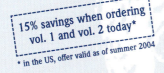

15% savings when ordering vol. 1 and vol. 2 today*

* in the US, offer valid as of summer 2004

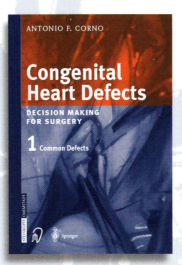

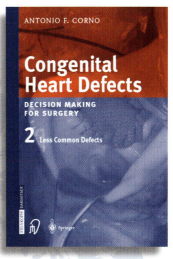

August 2003. 159 pages. 296 illustr. Hardbound EUR 119,95; US$ 129.00* ISBN 3-7985-1415-1

Summer 2004. app. 180 pages. 280 illustr. Hardbound EUR 119,95; US$ 129.00* ISBN 3-7985-1423-2

Table of Contents

STEINKOPFF DARMSTADT

Available in book stores or at STEINKOPFF Verlag • Fax: +49-6151-82899-40 • E-Mail: info.steinkopff@springer.de

Printing and Binding: Stürtz AG, Würzburg